MEDITERRANEAN DIET

COOKBOOK

FOR BEGINNERS

A Complete and Balanced Diet:

365 Days of Quick and Easy Recipes.

A Smart 28-Day Meal Plan For Healthy Eating.

GRACE M. WILLIAMSON

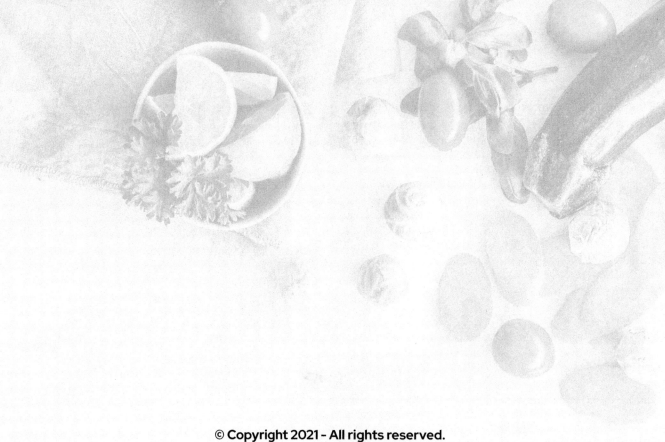

TABLE OF CONTENTS

INTRODUCTION

The Mediterranean diet is not new; it is one of the healthiest diets you can adopt. This diet is based on the regular eating patterns of those living in the Mediterranean regions such as Greece, Italy, and Spain. The protocols recommended by this diet are quite simple. It is essentially a plant-based diet that consists of heart-healthy fats and plenty of seafood. Calling it a "diet" is not entirely right, because it is more like a way of living. This diet encourages you to make good food choices and increases your consumption of fresh vegetables, fruits, whole grains, nuts and seeds, herbs and spices, legumes, and naturally fatty seafood. The Mediterranean diet is incredibly easy to follow and can be customized to suit your lifestyle. All you need to do is become conscious about your food choices. Yes, it is as simple as that!

In this book, you will learn about the origins of the well-balanced Mediterranean diet, the benefits it offers, dietary protocols, a detailed food list, and steps to get started. This book also includes tried and tested suggestions to accelerate your progress with the Mediterranean diet. Once you understand more about the diet, you can explore the different recipes provided in this book. All the recipes included are divided into different categories for your convenience. This book also includes a well-structured meal plan making it easy for you to get started with this diet.

Even if you are a novice, the recipes given in this book will make cooking quite easy. All you need to do is simply gather the required ingredients, choose a recipe, and follow the instructions. These are the only steps you need to follow to cook delicious, quick, and healthy meals within no time.

So, are you excited to learn about the Mediterranean diet? If yes, let's get started immediately!

AT THE END OF THE BOOK YOU'LL RECEIVE A GIFT!

WANT MORE RECIPES?

VISIT MY WEBSITE AND SIGN UP TO OUR NEWSLETTER TO KEEP UP TO DATE ON MANY NEW RECIPES

YOU CAN DOWNLOAD THIS FOOD LIST HERE TO PRINT IT OUT AND TAKE IT WITH YOU.

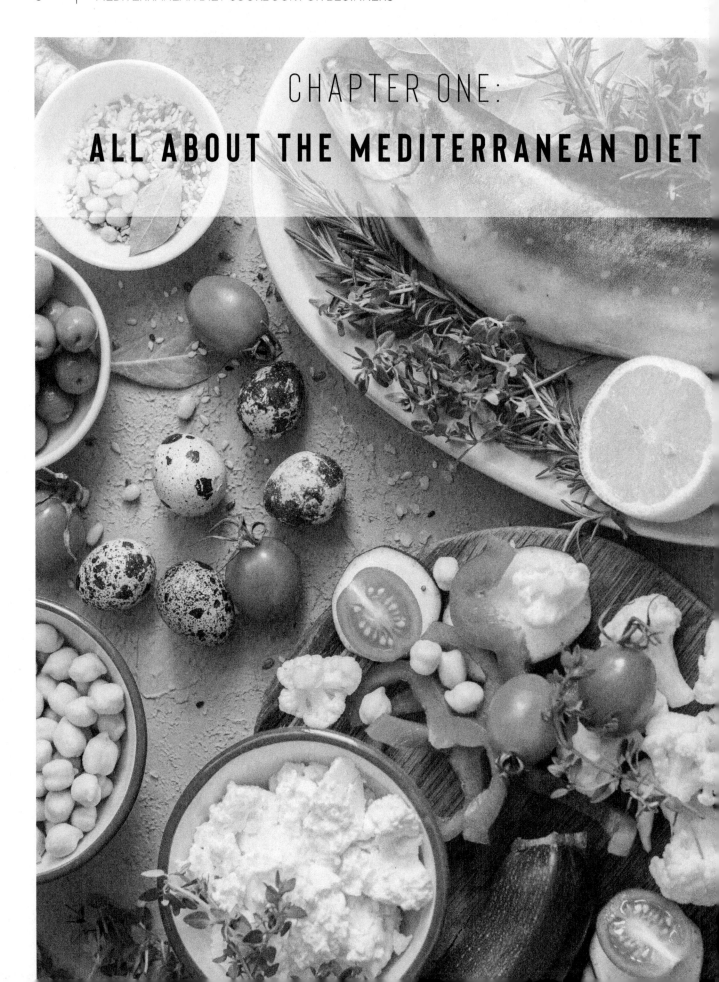

CHAPTER ONE:

ALL ABOUT THE MEDITERRANEAN DIET

The health benefits of the Mediterranean diet were first observed by Dr. Ancle Keys and his colleagues. During the 1950s and 1960s, Dr. Keys formed a hypothesis that those residing in the Mediterranean region were healthier when compared to others, especially compared to those in the Western Hemisphere. He associated these health benefits with the diet that those who live there follow. The coast of the Mediterranean Sea has 18 countries: Greece, Cyprus, Israel, Syria, Lebanon, Malta, southern France, Italy, Croatia, Bosnia, Spain, Turkey, Morocco, Algeria, Libya, Tunisia, Albania, and Egypt.

Despite the wide cultural diversity in these countries, their cuisine is quite similar. A commonality between the cuisines of all these regions is their reliance on fresh ingredients. The diet in these regions is typically a plant-based diet rich in seafood and plenty of olive oil. Temperature, climatic conditions, and location are some of the topographical factors responsible for making the cuisine of the Mediterranean region unique. Another similarity between the cuisine of these countries is the use of bold and flavorful spices and herbs, which complement and enhance the flavor of all the fresh ingredients used. This forms the basis of the Mediterranean diet.

A typical Mediterranean meal is well-balanced, rich in nutrients, flavors, colors, and textures. Whether it is a fresh filet of salmon served with a handful of salad leaves, crunchy nuts drizzled with olive oil and crumbled cheese, or a plate of figs topped with Greek yogurt and honey, the Mediterranean diet is rich in flavors. Unlike most fad diets, this is not restrictive by any means. If anything, the Mediterranean diet includes a variety of plant-based foods, seafood, and dietary fats.

The Mediterranean diet is not a low-fat or a low-carb diet. Instead, it is a well-balanced eating pattern that includes all the macro and micronutrients your body needs. It is devoid of processed and pre-packaged foods that dominate the typical Western diet such as processed meats, unhealthy carbs and sugars, and harmful trans fats. Instead, it shifts your focus to nutrient-dense ingredients your body needs to function efficiently. Even though it is a predominantly plant-based diet, it is not strictly vegetarian. It includes different types of naturally fatty fish, seafood, poultry, and limited amounts of red meat.

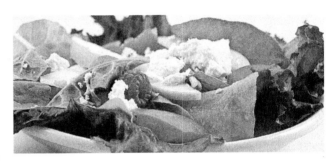

An important part of the Mediterranean diet is that it is a lifestyle and not just a diet. The Mediterranean culture is a celebration of food and people. It is about sharing meals with your loved ones and savoring food instead of mindless eating. Another characteristic of this diet is that it includes red wine! Yes, you read that right! Having a glass of red wine with a Mediterranean meal is quite common. The antioxidants present in red wine are good for your health. But, as with anything else in life, there needs to be moderation. This Mediterranean lifestyle doesn't promote leading a sedentary life, and instead, encourages you to engage in some form of physical activity or another. When you put all these factors together, the Mediterranean lifestyle is a great way to improve your physical and mental health.

Myths About the Mediterranean Diet

These days, any information is just a click away, but this easy access to information comes with its own set of problems. For instance, the spread of misinformation is quite high. Before you learn more about this diet, it is important to let go of certain misconceptions and myths associated with the Mediterranean diet.

Myth #1: The Mediterranean Diet Applies Only to the Mediterranean Region

This is one of the most common myths associated with this diet. Remember, it is based on the eating patterns of those residing in the Mediterranean region. If you take a moment and think about it, there's no reason to believe you cannot follow this diet as well. It is predominantly a plant-based diet that encourages the consumption of wholesome vegetables, fruits, legumes, whole grains, plenty of seafood, and poultry. All the food prescribed by this diet can be found anywhere and you can easily customize the meals according to your taste and preferences.

Myth #2: The Mediterranean Diet Is a High-Fat Diet

Most of us wrongly demonize fats and blame them for the steadily increasing rates of obesity and chronic illnesses. Well, it turns out we are all wrong. The actual culprits responsible for these conditions are carbs and sugars. The Mediterranean diet increases your consumption of healthy dietary fats instead of the unhealthy ones present in processed and packaged ingredients. This diet encourages your consumption of healthy fats while curbing the consumption of all unhealthy ones. The monounsaturated and polyunsaturated fats present in this diet are good for heart health and also reduces cholesterol levels. So, stop being scared of fats. Instead, embrace the Mediterranean diet to obtain all the different benefits it offers.

Myth #3: This Diet is All About Pasta, Cheese, and Pizza

The Mediterranean cuisine is extremely diverse and is not confined to pasta, pizza, or cheese. As mentioned, there are 18 countries in the Mediterranean region. This diet shifts your attention toward healthy and wholesome plant-based foods instead of getting stuck consuming unhealthy carbs and nutrient-devoid meals. The Mediterranean diet is not restricted to pizza, bread, or pasta. A typical Mediterranean meal contains plenty of vegetables, a small portion of fish or lean animal protein, and a small serving of carbs. This diet ensures your body gets all the macro and micronutrients it needs to function efficiently.

Myth #4: It Is Incredibly Difficult to Follow

The Mediterranean diet is synonymous with a healthy eating plan. It might increase your consumption of certain foods while restricting others, but all the foods included in this diet are nutritious. It encourages you to depend more on home-cooked meals instead of ordering in or consuming pre-cooked and processed meals. Most of us have unwittingly become accustomed to relying heavily on both these options when it comes to fulfilling our daily food requirements. Unfortunately, all this is undesirable. Once you shift to the Mediterranean diet, you will notice a significant reduction in your monthly food bills, especially when you start to regularly cook at home.

Myth #5: Drink Wine Freely

When it comes to the Mediterranean diet, or any other diet for that matter, moderation is important. An important characteristic of this diet is that it lets you consume the occasional glass of red wine. Red wine is good for your health because it is rich in antioxidants that are believed to strengthen cardiovascular function. If one glass of red wine is good, then 3 or 4 must be much better, right? This is nothing more than a misconception. Let go of this notion and stick to the food list discussed in subsequent chapters.

The Mediterranean diet helps to reduce the risk of diabetes, coronary diseases, and tackle inflammation while promoting weight loss and maintenance, and improves your cognitive health. By understanding the popular misconceptions and their associated facts, you'll be better equipped to shift to this diet.

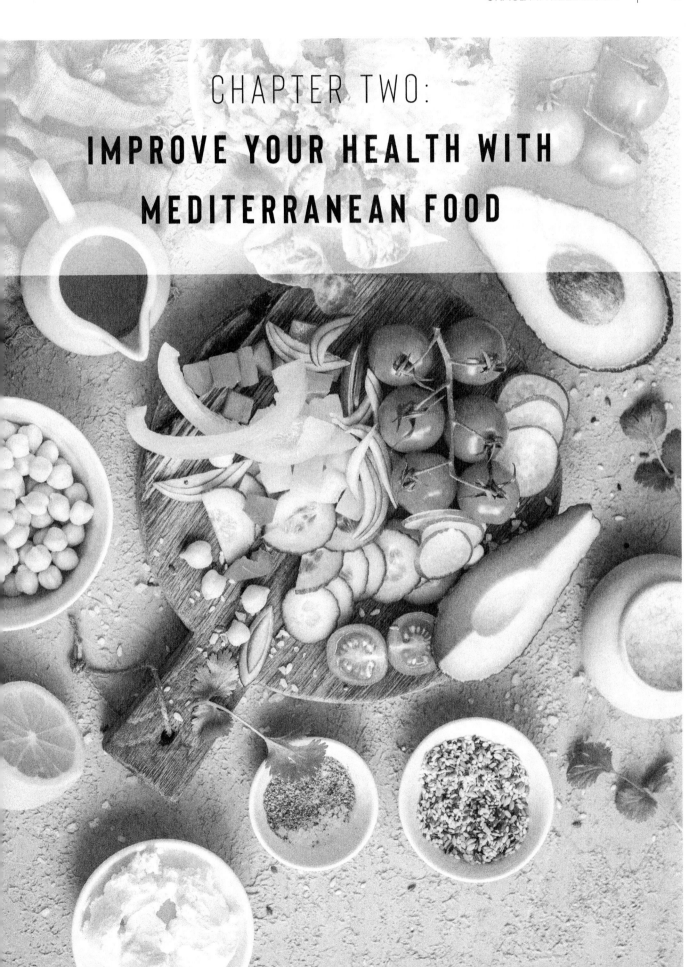

CHAPTER TWO:
IMPROVE YOUR HEALTH WITH MEDITERRANEAN FOOD

Whether you want to lose weight, lead a healthy life, or reduce the risk of any chronic health conditions, the Mediterranean diet will help. In this section, we will look at all the different benefits associated with the diet.

Improve Cardiovascular Health

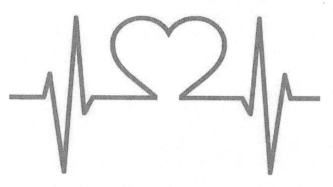

The Mediterranean diet is rich in Omega 3 fatty acids which are associated with better heart health. One of the most common ingredients used in the Mediterranean diet is olive oil. It is rich in alpha-linolenic acid (ALA) necessary for improving your cardiovascular health. The Mediterranean diet also increases your consumption of healthy and wholesome ingredients instead of processed foods that are filled with empty calories. An important benefit of olive oil is that it reduces hypertension. The nitric oxide produced by olive oil ensures that your arteries are dilated and there is no arterial plaque. Arterial plaque increases the risk of cardiovascular disorders including strokes.

Another important benefit of the healthy fatty acids included in this diet is that they reduce inflammation. According to a study conducted by Giuseppe Grosso et al. (2017), the Mediterranean diet is believed to improve coronary health. In a 5-year study conducted by Ramon Estruch et al. (2013), 7,000 men and women in Spain with a high risk of cardiovascular diseases were asked to follow a Mediterranean diet. The researchers noticed those who followed this diet had a 30% lower risk of developing coronary diseases when compared to others. According to a study undertaken by Katherine E. Paterson et al. (2018), the Mediterranean diet can reduce the risk of strokes. The researchers of this study noticed the risk of strokes in participants reduced by 20% in women, even ones with a high risk of stroke, by following the Mediterranean diet.

When you put all these factors together and look at the supporting evidence, it becomes obvious the Mediterranean diet is a great way to improve your cardiovascular health.

Improves Cognitive Health

Cognitive health, including your memory and thinking skills, tends to decrease with age. The brain is an incredibly complex organ responsible for all your functions. It is also a very hungry organ. It needs a constant supply of oxygen and nutrients derived from the bloodstream. If you have any existing problems with vascular health or an increased risk of cardiovascular disorders, this increases the risk of developing any issues associated with your cognitive health. Usually, it presents itself as cognitive decline associated with degenerative disorders such as Alzheimer's and Parkinson's.

According to a study conducted by Roy J. Hardman et al. (2016), following a Mediterranean diet can improve cognitive functioning, slow down cognitive decline, and even reduce the risk of developing Alzheimer's. These findings were backed by another study undertaken by Valentina Berti et al. (2018). The cognitive health benefits associated with this diet are due to the consumption of healthy fats including olive oil, nuts, and other anti-inflammatory foods. These wholesome ingredients help counteract the harmful effects of inflammation associated with a poor diet.

Promotes Weight Loss and Maintenance

The Mediterranean diet increases your intake of healthy fats and proteins while reducing unhealthy carb consumption. By including naturally healthy and fatty oils such as Omega 3 fatty acids from seafood, foods rich in dietary fiber, and a variety of probiotics, your satiety levels automatically increase. If your hunger is satiated, it automatically reduces hunger pangs. This, in turn, makes it easier to practice portion control without feeling restricted.

A typical Western diet is rich in processed and pre-packaged ingredients. Most of us are guilty of making unhealthy food choices daily. If you take a moment and think about it, different foods have different satiety levels. For instance, eating a bag of chips or cookies might satiate your hunger initially, but you will feel hungry within an hour or two. On the other hand, if you eat a healthy bowl of salad filled with protein, you will not feel hungry for longer. Why does this happen? This is because plant-based foods are rich in dietary fiber that increases your satiety levels. If your hunger is satiated, the urge to binge on unhealthy foods automatically reduces.

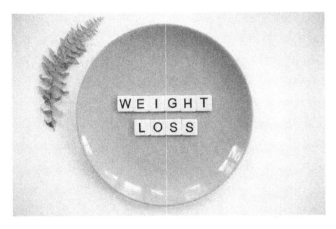

Instead of counting every calorie you consume, the idea of the Mediterranean diet is to choose healthy and nutrient-dense ingredients. Because of this, your calorie intake automatically decreases. Maintaining a calorie deficit becomes easier. A calorie deficit occurs when your calorie expenditure is more than calorie intake. According to a study conducted by Iris Shai et al. (2008), a diet rich in extra-virgin olive oil promotes weight loss even without calorie restriction. If weight loss is your priority, combining the Mediterranean diet with calorie restriction and exercise can further enhance weight loss and maintenance.

Reduces the Risk of Type-2 Diabetes

Diabetes is a metabolic disorder characterized by high levels of blood sugar or limited levels of insulin in the bloodstream. Your body requires a pancreatic enzyme known as insulin, which is responsible for regulating your blood sugar levels. Your body cannot process glucose by itself and requires insulin to convert it into usable energy molecules. Type 2 diabetes is a steadily growing health problem across the globe. It's characterized by a condition where your body cannot produce the insulin required to process glucose. It, in turn, increases blood sugar levels. The most common risk factors associated with developing diabetes are a high sugar diet, unhealthy lifestyle, stress, and obesity. If your diet is rich in processed and packaged food, greasy and fatty fried foods, and other unhealthy ingredients, the risk of diabetes increases. So, the best thing you can do right now is to counteract this condition by shifting to a healthy and wholesome diet devoid of processed foods.

According to the research conducted by Jordi Salas-Salvado et al. (2011), following a Mediterranean diet can reduce the risk of type-2 diabetes. The Mediterranean diet increases your consumption of wholesome vegetables, fruits, legumes, whole grains, healthy fats, and seafood. According to the research conducted by Olubukola Ajala et al. (2013), the Mediterranean diet promotes the regulation of blood sugar levels when compared to a low-carb or a high-protein diet.

Reduces Inflammation

Your immune system is responsible for protecting your body from pathogens and foreign invaders such as disease-causing microorganisms. The first line of defense of the immune system is inflammation. In regulated amounts, inflammation is not only desirable but is important for maintaining your health and is a sign of a well-functioning immune system. Unfortunately, if inflammation levels are left unregulated, they become problematic and trigger a variety of painful conditions including rheumatoid arthritis. Certain foods support the function of the immune system while others trigger inflammation. Some common foods that trigger inflammation include red meats, processed foods, processed meats, sugars, harmful carbs, and unhealthy hydrogenated oils and trans fats. The Mediterranean diet is devoid of all these harmful ingredients. Therefore, it can reduce inflammation. The healthy dietary fats and complex carbs suggested by this diet tackle inflammation.

According to the research conducted by Giuseppe Grosso et al. (2017), the anti-inflammatory omega-3 fatty acids present in naturally fatty seafood and olive oil can reduce the painful symptoms of arthritis. The anti-inflammatory fatty acids reverse inflammation and in turn, reduce symptoms associated with conditions triggered by inflammation such as rheumatoid arthritis.

The Mediterranean diet increases your intake of wholesome vegetables and fruits rich in a variety of antioxidants. These antioxidants help neutralize inflammation and reduce the risk associated with inflammatory conditions. Leading causes of inflammation include a poor diet and leading a sedentary lifestyle. By shifting to this diet, you can successfully reverse inflammation while strengthening the functioning of your immune system.

Reduces the Risk of Certain Types of Cancer

Consuming a tired rich in fiber, antioxidants, polyphenols, and healthy Omega 6 and Omega 3 fatty acids combats and prevents the biological mechanisms associated with developing cancer. While following the Mediterranean diet, you can easily obtain all these essential nutrients. A plant-based diet includes wholesome vegetable fruits and whole grains. These ingredients promote your body's ability to fight cancer by providing the required antioxidants. As mentioned, antioxidants reduce any damage caused to the DNA reducing the risk of cell mutation. Antioxidants also reduce the levels of inflammation. A combination of these factors is believed to reduce the risk of certain types of cancer. According to a meta-analysis undertaken by Lukas Scwingshackl et al. (2017), following the Mediterranean diet can reduce the risk of colorectal and breast cancer. According to a study conducted by Estefania Toledo et al. (2015), the Mediterranean diet reduces the risk of breast cancer in women by 62% when compared to those following a low-fat diet.

Helps Ease Depression

Your diet plays a significant role in your mental well-being. Yes, what you eat affects how you feel. If you take a moment to think, it makes sense. How do you feel after a heavy meal? Chances are you feel quite tired, lethargic, and drowsy. On the other hand, how do you feel after a light meal of a super salad? You will feel energetic!

According to an analysis of observational studies undertaken by Camille Lassale et al. (2019), the Mediterranean diet can reduce the risk of depression when compared to pro-inflammatory diets. The regular Western diet is a pro-inflammatory diet characterized by high levels of trans fats, refined sugars and carbs, processed meats, and empty calories.

Avoiding foods that harm your cognitive health and increasing the intake of antioxidants has a positive effect on your overall mood.

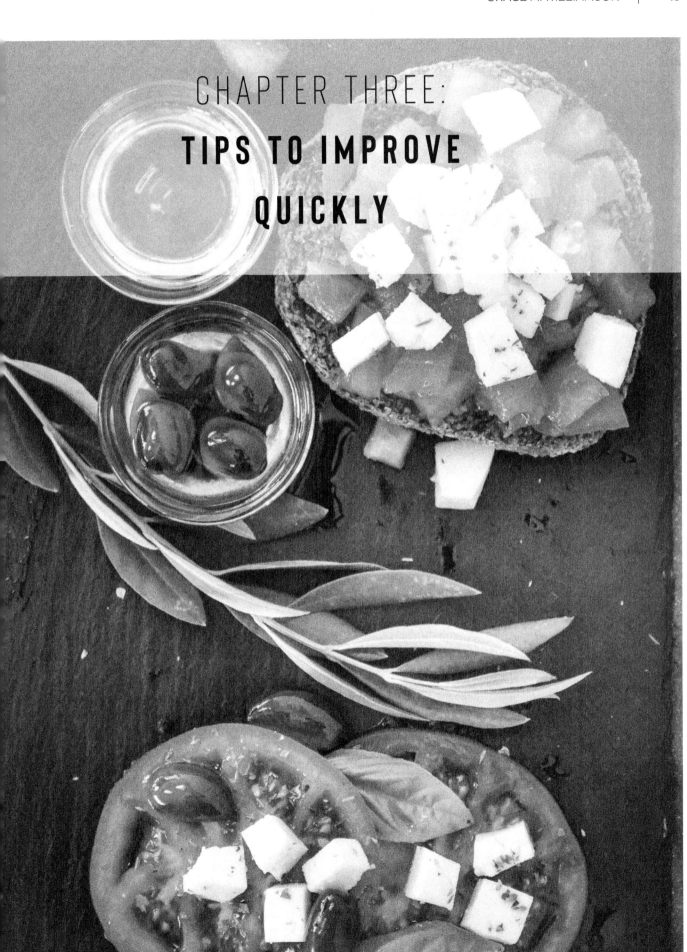

CHAPTER THREE:
TIPS TO IMPROVE QUICKLY

The Mediterranean diet is extremely healthy and easy to follow. What if there was something else you can do to accelerate your progress while following this diet? Yes, you read it right. It is possible to accelerate the result obtained from this diet. In this chapter, you learn about the common mistakes beginners make and how to avoid them, and several tips to enhance the overall benefits offered by the diet.

Tips to Follow

In this section, you will learn about simple tips you can use to make things easier while following the Mediterranean diet.

Cook at Home

Start cooking at home as much as you possibly can. Cooking is not a difficult task. Now that you are armed with all the different recipes given in this book, cooking well becomes a breeze. Simply stock the pantry with the required ingredients, select a recipe that appeals to you, and follow the simple instructions. These are the only steps involved to cook delicious meals. Cooking becomes even easier if you practice meal prep over the weekend and start batch cooking. When you cook the meals at home, your relationship with food will improve. It makes you more conscious of everything you are eating. Apart from this, it gives you complete control over the quality of ingredients used and the portions too.

Practice Mindful Eating

Learn to savor every morsel you consume. A lot of effort went into not only growing the produce you are eating, but in cooking it too. It is important to enjoy the fruits of your labor. Instead of watching TV, working, or checking emails, keep all these gadgets away and focus only on the food you are eating. Eating meals with your loved ones is also a great way to practice mindful eating. Whenever you eat, learn to savor the taste, aroma, texture, and flavors. When you start paying attention to all this, you automatically become conscious of how much you are eating. When you are watching something on TV, chances are that you end up overeating without even realizing it. By shifting your attention to the present, paying attention to how much we eat becomes easy.

When you eat slowly, it gives you a better opportunity to chew the food thoroughly before swallowing. This simple practice promotes your body's ability to digest and absorb nutrients present in the food you eat.

Plan All Meals

Make it a point to eat three healthy, wholesome, and well-rounded meals daily. Yes, eating breakfast is a part of the Mediterranean way of living. If you are used to skipping breakfast, it's time to make some changes. A simple way to increase your chances of following this diet without giving in to the temptation of eating out or depending on pre-packaged meals is through meal planning. Take some time over the weekend, think about all the different meals you want to eat, and start planning. Meal planning ensures plenty of variety is incorporated into your usual diet. It is also a great way to reduce the cooking time during the week. Instead of wasting your precious resources thinking about what your next meal should be, start planning. Meal planning is also important for grocery shopping. Don't forget to use the sample meal plan discussed in this book to make things easier. Once you get into the groove of following the Mediterranean diet, you can create your own meal plans too.

Ration Your Portions

Even though the Mediterranean diet doesn't encourage calorie counting, exercising portion control is important. This reduces the risk of overeating while ensuring your body gets its daily dose of essential nutrients. As a rule of thumb, fill up on lean protein, dietary fiber, and complex carbs to ensure you receive the daily dose of nutrients. Whether it is weighing the portions or storing them in specific containers, practicing portion control is important.

Clean Your Pantry

Before you start this diet, spend some time and carefully go through all the ingredients you have at home. Not just ingredients, but the different food items too. If there is anything that doesn't fit the Mediterranean eating pattern, get rid of it. Think of it as spring-cleaning for the kitchen. Out of sight out of mind is a great way to deal with temptations. This is especially true if you have plenty of refined and processed foods at home such as chips, cookies, chocolate, ice creams, and so on. Once you have cleared the pantry, you'll have sufficient place to accommodate Mediterranean diet-friendly ingredients.

Grocery Shopping

Once you are aware of your meal plan, it automatically becomes easier to determine the groceries you will need. Whenever you go to the supermarket, carry the grocery list with you. Go through the Mediterranean food list discussed in previous chapters to create a shopping list and stick to it. In the previous step, it was mentioned you need to clean the pantry, now it's time to restock it with all Mediterranean diet ingredients.

Choose Local and Seasonal Produce

Whenever possible, opt for seasonal and locally produced ingredients. These are wholesome and more nutritious. Not to mention, they are also relatively low in cost when compared to other ingredients. Perhaps visit the local farmer's market or even a farm, if there is any nearby. It will give you a better idea of where your produce comes from.

Set a Food Budget

If you are worried following the Mediterranean diet will burn a hole in your pocket, you need to think again. As mentioned previously, believing the Mediterranean diet to be expensive is nothing more than a myth. When it comes to following a diet, your food choices play a crucial role. The simplest way to ensure you don't go overboard or spend too much on the diet by setting a food budget. At the start of the month, create a meal plan, and make a list of all the ingredients you will need. Add a little buffer to it and you have your food budget. Ensure you do not exceed this. Well, it's not just your body, even your bank balance will be grateful for this diet.

Meal Prep Is Your Friend

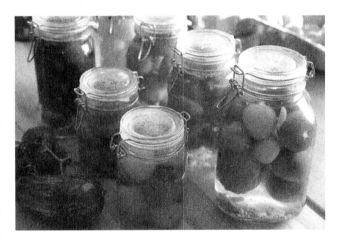

Meal prepping essentially means doing the required prep for a meal before you start cooking. Think of it as laying down the groundwork. It includes simple tasks such as portioning the protein, chopping vegetables, making sauces, cooking the meat, and so on. Cooking becomes easy when all the meal prep is ready. It hardly takes an hour or two over the weekend to meal prep for a week. Before you start, ensure you have a meal plan place. Meal prep is also a great way to practice portion control. When you look at a meal plan, you will realize certain ingredients are overlapping. Also, ingredients used in a specific meal can be repurposed for other meals.

Another advantage is it gives you a chance to batch cook. If there is a specific recipe you like or enjoy, cook multiple portions of it and store it for later. Whether it is a sauce, curry, broth, soup, or a casserole, you can batch cook these recipes. Cooking during the week becomes a breeze when the basic prep is done.

Never Leave the Home Hungry

Make it a point to never leave your home hungry. This increases the risk of temptations. If you are hungry, you will want to eat something. If your hunger is satiated, the chances of any hunger pangs tempting you when will reduce automatically. If not, you can always carry some snacks with you. It becomes easier to stick to this diet when you are not hungry. Also, hunger is a primary reason why a lot of people give up on diets. So, pay attention to your body's hunger cues.

Make Healthy Snacks

Make a few healthy Mediterranean diet-friendly snacks at home. Whether it is roasted chickpeas, kale chips, or baked pita strips, making some healthy snacks is not time-consuming. It also ensures you are following the diet regardless of where you are. Whether you're going to work or traveling, carry some of these snacks with you at all times. All it takes is a little creativity and cooking becomes quite easy. Making snacks at home is cost-effective and incredibly healthy because it gives you complete control over the quality of ingredients used and the portion size too.

Fill Up on Healthy Foods

While following any diet, there will be days when you feel like binging on something unhealthy. If you are craving something sweet, remind yourself you can eat it later after you finished your daily portion of protein, complex carbs, dietary fats, and fiber. Chances are, by the time you have filled up on these foods, you will no longer be hungry or have any space for the sweet treat you

were craving. This is a great technique that reduces any feelings of deprivation while ensuring your body gets all the nourishment it needs.

Don't Forget to Exercise

An important aspect of the Mediterranean lifestyle is to be active. So, do not forget to exercise. It becomes easier to attain and maintain your weight loss goals when exercise is a part of your daily routine. Exercising regularly is good for your mental health too. It is not only a great stress buster but improves the production of feel-good hormones.

You don't have to incorporate all these suggestions at once. Start with one or two tips and incorporate them into your daily routine. Once they become a part of your routine, you can work on other tips. It's quite easy to get overwhelmed when you look at the list of things that need to be done. Well, the good news is, there's no rush. You can take your time and pace yourself.

Mistakes to Avoid

Understanding how the Mediterranean diet works are important if you want to increase your chances of success. Learning about all the foods you can and cannot eat will make it easy to follow the diet. However, there are certain common mistakes beginners make while transitioning to this diet. In this section, let's look at these mistakes and how you can avoid them.

Drastically Increasing Your Intake of Grains And Cereals

The Mediterranean diet includes healthy servings of different grains and cereals. Your consumption of grains and cereals depends on your level of physical activity. If you are leading a sedentary lifestyle, concentrate on adding some exercise to your daily routine. Whole grains and cereals are rich in carbs and unless your body gets the exercise it needs, consuming too many carbs is seldom desirable. Remember, the Mediterranean diet is not just about eating plenty of pasta or bread. Instead, it is about consuming well-balanced meals that include all the different types of nutrients your body needs.

Not Practicing Portion Control

The Mediterranean diet does not include any restrictive calorie requirement. You don't have to count every calorie present in every morsel you eat. It is important to pay attention to the portions you consume. This is especially true when you are talking about healthy fats such as olive oil and nuts. You don't have to place any hard limits on your daily intake of vegetables. However, if you eat too many seeds and nuts, dairy products, and red meat, it doesn't make any sense. One important rule of following the Mediterranean diet is to practice the idea of moderation. Ensure that every meal you consume includes carbohydrates, proteins, dietary fats, and dietary fiber.

Not Paying Attention to The Cheese You Consume

Dairy is not a major food group when it comes to the Mediterranean diet. It is important for a healthy diet, but only in limited amounts. Cheese is never the star in any Mediterranean meal. Instead, it is incorporated into salad dressings or used as a topping. Pay attention to the dietary choices you make. You can consume Greek yogurt, provided it is the unsweetened variety. Choosing artificially flavored yogurt is not good for your health. Most of the prepackaged yogurts available on the market these days include added sugar and preservatives. Unsweetened Greek yogurt topped with some fresh fruits and nuts is a healthy dessert while artificially flavored yogurt is rich in calories or nothing else.

Not Eating Sufficient Seafood

Make it a point to consume seafood at least twice a week. Even though it is a predominantly plant-based diet, it is not a vegetarian diet. You need to consume naturally fatty fish and seafood. The Omega 3 fatty acids present in fish and shellfish are good for your brain and body alike. So, start increasing your intake of seafood. Whenever possible, opt for fish caught in the wild instead of the factory-farmed variants.

Skipping Meals

If you are trying to lose weight or maintain it, it can be quite tempting to skip meals. As a rule of thumb, avoid skipping meals. It is okay to not eat when you are not hungry. Start paying attention to your body's hunger cues. Following the diet becomes difficult if you start skipping meals. Unless you eat healthy and wholesome meals, you will not get the desired nutrition. Skipping meals does more harm than good.

If you are exercising, ensure you refuel afterward. Exercising intensively and skipping meals will shift your body into starvation mode. Once in this mode, your body stops burning fats and instead, starts hoarding them. This is undesirable if weight loss is your priority.

Drinking Too Much Wine

Even though this diet lets you drink red wine, do not go overboard. Drinking too much wine and not drinking sufficient water is a recipe for disaster. Alcohol might not be a staple of the Mediterranean eating style, but in limited amounts, it is helpful. Red wine, especially the dry varieties, is the only ideal choice of alcohol. You cannot drink white wine, tequila, gin, beer, or any other form of alcohol and believe it's all the same. Even though red wine is good for you, don't forget the rule about moderation. You can have a glass of red wine with your meals, but don't forget to drink sufficient water at the same time. Staying hydrated is crucial if you want to follow this diet or any other diet for that matter.

Don't Limit Flavors

Let go of any conceptions that diet food is bland or flavorless. Do not restrict yourself when it comes to using herbs and spices. Instead of depending on salt to flavor your meals, include a variety of herbs and spices. It is important to ensure you consume healthy and flavorful meals. If you eat the same food daily, sticking to this diet will become boring and incredibly difficult. Similarly, eating bland food will also make things difficult. The Mediterranean diet is a celebration of produce. Get into the spirit of the Mediterranean way of living by adding bold and exciting flavors to all the meals you consume.

Do Not Use Processed Foods as a Substitute

A healthy shortcut is acceptable, but relying on processed foods is not a good idea. Depending on that instant box of couscous is a bad idea. Artificial sweeteners, chemical additives, preservatives, unhealthy trans fats, and refined carbs are present in all different processed foods. So, stay away from them. You can look for healthy shortcuts such as using canned beans when you are pressed for time. If you want to follow this diet, concentrate on making healthy food choices. Avoid using fast food as a shortcut because it is a bad choice in the long run. The idea of this diet is to increase your intake of wholesome and fresh ingredients while reducing dependence on unhealthy foods. Concentrate on attaining this goal and your nutrient intake will automatically increase full stock

Many believe that experience is the best teacher. After all, when you make a mistake, it is a valuable learning opportunity. Well, you don't necessarily have to keep making mistakes to learn those lessons. There's a lot to learn from the mistakes that others make and their experience. By avoiding the simple mistakes suggested in the section, you can increase your chances of success. Avoiding these mistakes will make it easier to follow the Mediterranean diet and transform it into a sustainable lifestyle.

Tips to Stay Motivated

Motivation is the internal desire that keeps you going even when you don't want to. You can do the right thing even when you don't feel like it. Without motivation,

getting anything done in life will become quite difficult. It is essentially the fuel that helps attain your goals despite any obstacles or challenges you face. It is an incredibly important part of all aspects of life and your diet is not an exception. Usually, whenever you try something new, chances are you are quite excited during an initial couple of days. After a while, the excitement and novelty fade away and your motivation levels reduce. There will be situations when your motivation levels falter, especially after a setback or a challenge. It is important to maintain your motivation levels because the Mediterranean diet is a long-term solution. It is a lifestyle choice and not just a short-term diet. Unless you are motivated from the inside, shifting to this lifestyle will become unnecessarily difficult.

One of the simplest ways to stay motivated is by establishing realistic and relevant goals for yourself. You need to set small, measurable, and time-bound goals. It essentially means vague goals are nothing more than a recipe for disaster and appointment. For instance, a goal such as, "I want to lose weight," is quite vague. On the other hand, a goal such as, "I want to lose 10 pounds within 3 months," is extremely specific. It not only tells you what you want to do but the time frame within which you should attain it. It is important to establish time-bound goals because if you don't have a time limit, the chances of procrastination increase.

Apart from setting goals, there are different things you can do to maintain your motivation levels. In this section, let's look at some helpful tips for staying motivated.

Do Not Rush Into It

It can be quite tempting to rush into a diet. Well, it is not a good idea. Instead, take some time and plan how you want to go about it. Remember, you need to shop for groceries, plan the meals, and determine how you want to go about this diet. Unless you complete all these steps, the chances of giving up on it increase. Since you are in it for the long run, do not rush into it.

Learn to be patient if you want to follow this diet. Making a lifestyle change is not something that happens overnight. Also, it will take a while before you can see some results. In the meanwhile, it is important to not give up on the diet. Follow this diet for at least 4 weeks to see a positive change. Learn to be patient with yourself and trust this diet. After all, you did not gain those extra pounds overnight, and losing them overnight is nothing but impractical. It is not a crash diet and is a healthy lifestyle change.

While following the diet, you will hit a weight loss plateau. This is not only common, but you should expect it too. A weight-loss plateau occurs when you stop losing weight despite following the diet and exercising regularly. When you hit this plateau, it is important to reconsider your diet and change your exercise routine a little. For instance, reducing the carbohydrate intake while increasing protein consumption and changing the form of exercise can help overcome this plateau. It is a process of trial and error. So, be patient and don't be in a hurry.

Change Your Mindset

Don't discount the importance of mindset while following a diet. If you believe the diet is restrictive or depriving you of foods you enjoy, following it will become tricky. On the other hand, concentrating on all the foods you can eat creates a positive mindset. Let go of any reservations, biases, and misconceptions about it. Approach this diet with an open mind and you will be pleasantly surprised.

Prepare for Setbacks

Setbacks are not only common, but you should expect them too. You cannot succeed without dealing with a few setbacks. There will be times when you give in to your temptations and eat something you know you're not supposed to. In such instances, understand that it is okay. If you have slipped up, pick yourself up and get back to the routine from the following day. It

is okay to indulge yourself. However, it's not okay to view all this as a failure. Create a plan of action to deal with such setbacks. For instance, if you had a packet of chips, restrict yourself to it and don't go overboard. Every setback is an isolated incident. Do not treat it as a general pattern. Don't give up on the diet and get back to it from the following day.

Let Go of Any Notions of Perfection

Let go of an all-or-nothing attitude. If you want to follow this diet and maintain the results, you should not hold on to any notions of perfection. Perfection is nothing more than a mirage. If you keep chasing it, you are setting yourself up for disappointment. A perfectionist attitude can quickly turn a setback into a failure. It also prevents you from acknowledging all the efforts you make. It is better to concentrate on your efforts instead of the results during the initial stages.

As mentioned, you should not only prepare yourself for setbacks but expect them too. It is a human tendency to make mistakes. If you aim for perfection, it can prevent you from taking the first step itself. If you don't try, you will never know and with a perfectionist attitude, you will always be scared to get started. Another problem with this kind of thinking is you start viewing every setback as a failure. Even if you make a mistake, there is a specific lesson to be learned. Once you learn the lessons, you can move on and prevent them from occurring again.

Buddy Up

It becomes easier to follow a diet when you have a partner. Whether it is your spouse, family member, friend, or even an online friend, buddy up. When you know you are not alone, following the diet automatically becomes easier. Imagine, if you had someone else to plan the meals with, shop for groceries, and exercise together, everything would become fun and exciting. Your dieting partner can also give you the motivation on the days when you are running a little low on it.

Apart from a dieting buddy, you need to create a support system too. Before you start the diet, talk to your close friends, and family members about your reasons for following this diet and what you wish to achieve. They will act as your support system and step in on those days when your motivation levels are quite low. By creating an external source of accountability, the added pressure will ensure you are following the diet and are sticking to your commitment. When you know you are accountable to someone else, the motivation to follow through on your promise automatically increases.

Establish Rewards

It is quite easy to criticize yourself whenever you make a mistake. If you are quick to criticize, ensure you are acknowledging all the wins that come your way. As mentioned, following the Mediterranean way of living is an amalgamation of all the small steps you take daily. Every positive step you take is an achievement. Don't forget to celebrate them. Acknowledging and celebrating all your victories, whether they are big or small, gives you the motivation to keep going.

For instance, if one of your goals is to avoid junk food for a month, don't forget to reward yourself when you have attained it. The only thing you need to remember while establishing rewards is to not make them anything food-related. For instance, it does not make any sense if you reward yourself by eating a pint of ice cream after foregoing junk food for a month. All the effort you put in is automatically undone. Instead, treat yourself to simple rewards such as watching a movie, getting a manicure pedicure, or even buying something special for yourself.

Create a Maintenance Plan

Remember, the Mediterranean diet is not a short-term solution. Instead, think of it as a lifestyle change. It is not a fad diet that promises overnight results. Instead, is a tried and tested dietary regime that offers a variety of health benefits. If you want to follow it in the long run, you need a maintenance plan. A maintenance plan is a combination of a good dietary regime and healthy lifestyle changes. Some simple healthy lifestyle changes suggested by this diet include adding exercise to your daily routine and spending time with loved ones. When you make these changes, your overall quality of life will improve. So, it's not just your health that improves, but you feel better about yourself.

Maintain a Journal

Start maintaining a dietary journal. It's not just about tracking all the different food choices you make but make a note of all the changes you observe in yourself. Once you start following this diet and get accustomed to it, you will realize your energy levels are higher, you sleep better at night, and start enjoying food more than ever. These are all positive changes that cannot be measured. By maintaining a journal, you can make a note of it. On the days when your motivation levels are running a little low, check this journal and you will feel better.

Also, take a picture of yourself before you start this diet. Instead of concentrating solely on the weighing scale, look for physical changes. Whether it is a reduction in your waist circumference or an improvement in your energy levels. Or maybe your clothes start fitting you better. These changes cannot be measured. That said, you should not ignore them because they are small victories. Look for these non-scalable victories and celebrate them.

Start following all these simple suggestions daily to increase your motivation levels. When you are motivated from the inside, following this diet, in the long run, becomes quite simple. It also ensures you not only attain your health and weight loss goals but maintain the results too.

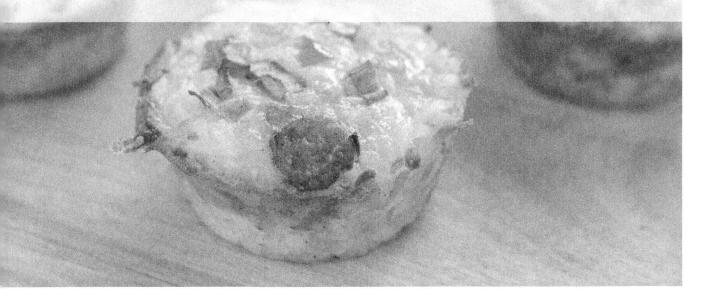

CHAPTER FOUR:
THE BEST RECIPES AND MEAL PLAN
TO START THE MEDITERRANEAN DIET

Calorie counting might sound restrictive and cumbersome, but is needed to ensure that you are not going to overeat. Also, by restricting your calorie intake, achieving and maintaining your weight loss and fitness goals becomes easier too. What more? Calorie counting is not complicated! In this chapter, you will discover a four-week meal plan and recipes to cook delicious and nutritious meals within a daily calorie limit of 1,500-1,600! If you want to further reduce your calorie intake, omitting one recipe from the daily meal plan helps. Maintaining a calorie deficit is needed for weight loss and maintenance.

If you are new to following a diet or counting calories, this chapter will make your life easier. All the recipes mention the calories they contain. Also, don't hesitate to experiment with the different recipes given here. Once you get the basic flavor combinations and pairings used in Mediterranean cuisine, cooking becomes exciting. You can also customize this sample meal plan according to your tastes and preferences.

NOTE: Before you decide to reduce or restrict your calorie intake, consult with your healthcare provider. Depending on your existing health and the fitness goals you want to achieve, your calorie requirements will also differ.

WEEK 1 - MONDAY

AVOCADO BREAKFAST SCRAMBLE (BREAKFAST)

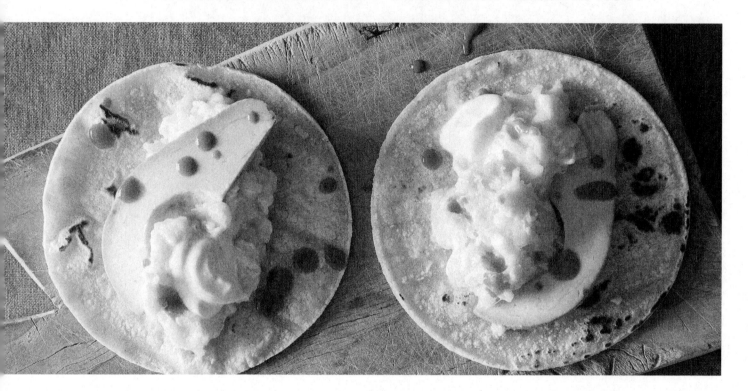

Number of servings:	Nutritional values per serving:				
1	Calories:	254	Carbohydrate: 16,05g	Protein:	10,99g
	Fat:	17,15g	Fiber: 3,44g		

Ingredients:

- 2 large eggs
- ½ avocado, peeled, pitted, sliced
- Juice of ½ lime
- ½ tablespoon butter, cubed
- Freshly cracked pepper to taste
- A small handful cherry or
- grape tomatoes, halved
- Salt to taste

Directions:

1. Add eggs, salt, and butter into a pan. Place the pan over medium low heat. Stir often and cook until the eggs are soft cooked.
2. Transfer the scrambled eggs on a plate. Scatter avocado and tomatoes over the eggs. Sprinkle salt, pepper, and lime juice on top and serve.

MINI OMELET MUFFINS (SNACK)

Number of servings:

2

Nutritional values per serving:
Two muffins

Calories:	370	**Carbohydrate:** 3,2g	**Protein:**	26g
Fat:	28g	**Fiber:** 2g		

Ingredients:

- 1–2 teaspoons olive oil
- ¼ cup skim milk or half and half
- 2 tablespoons grated
- cheddar cheese
- ½ cup chopped vegetables of your choice
- 1 teaspoon Italian seasoning
- 4 eggs
- Salt to taste

Directions:

1. You need to preheat your oven to 350°F.
2. As the oven is preheating, whisk eggs with milk, salt, and Italian seasoning.
3. Stir in cheddar cheese and vegetables.
4. Grease four ramekins with oil. Spoon the egg mixture into the ramekins.
5. Place the ramekins in a baking pan. Pour hot water all around the ramekins, up to about ½ the height of the ramekin.
6. Now place the ramekins along with the baking pan, in the oven and let it bake until it sets, about 30 minutes.
7. You can also make the omelets in a muffin pan. Place the muffin pan directly in the oven.

BLACK BEAN-QUINOA BUDDHA BOWL (LUNCH)

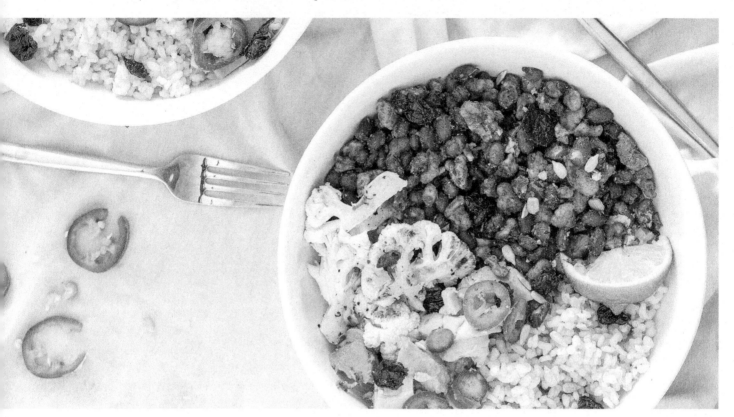

Number of servings:	**Nutritional values per serving:**		
2	**Calories:** 500	**Carbohydrate:** 74g	**Protein:** 20g
	Fat: 16g	**Fiber:** 20g	

Ingredients:

- 1½ cups cooked or canned black beans, rinsed, drained
- ½ cup hummus
- ½ medium avocado, peeled,

- pitted, diced
- ¼ cup chopped fresh cilantro
- 11/3 cups cooked quinoa

- 2 tablespoons lime juice
- 6 tablespoons pico de gallo

Directions:

1. Follow the instructions on the package of quinoa and cook quinoa. Measure out 11/3 cups of quinoa and add into a bowl. Add black beans and stir. Divide the mixture into two serving bowls.

2. To make dressing: Whisk together hummus and lime juice in a bowl. Add a little water if you want a thinner dressing.

3. Divide and drizzle the dressing over the bean mixture.

4. Place avocado and pico de gallo on top. Garnish with cilantro and serve.

GARLICKY MUSHROOM PENNE (DINNER)

Nutritional values per serving:

Number of servings:	Calories:	436	Carbohydrate:	59g	Protein:	18g
4	Fat:	12g	Fiber:	13g		

Ingredients:

For hummus:

- 1 can (14.5 ounces) chickpeas with its liquid
- 2 large cloves garlic, peeled, minced
- 4 teaspoons tahini
- Juice of a lemon

- Salt to taste
- 8.1 ounces whole wheat pasta
- 4 red onions, sliced
- Lemon juice to serve
- 2 teaspoons crumbled vegetable bouillon

- ½ teaspoon ground coriander
- 4 teaspoons olive oil
- 14 ounces mushrooms, roughly chopped
- ½ cup chopped parsley

Directions:

1. For hummus: Add chickpeas, lemon juice, garlic, tahini and salt into a blender and blend until most of it is smooth or slightly chunky with a few pieces of chickpeas.
2. Follow the directions on the package and cook the pasta.
3. Place a large nonstick pan or a wok over medium-high heat. Add oil. When the oil is heated, add onion and mushroom and cook until tender. Add vegetable bouillon and coriander and mix well.
4. Add pasta and toss well. Add hummus and toss lightly. Sprinkle some water if required.
5. Garnish with parsley and divide into plates. Drizzle some lemon juice on top and serve.

TUESDAY

SPRING GREEN FRITTATA (BREAKFAST)

Number of servings:

4

Nutritional values per serving:
One wedge

Calories:	214	**Carbohydrate:** 7,2g	**Protein:**	18,4g
Fat:	12,4g	**Fiber:** 1,7g		

Ingredients:

- 8 egg whites
- 4 eggs
- 4 tablespoons fat-free milk
- ¼ teaspoon black pepper
- 4 teaspoons olive oil
- ½ cup sliced green onions

- 2 cloves garlic, minced
- 2 teaspoons chopped chives
- ½ cup finely shredded Parmesan cheese
- 1 cup sliced asparagus (½

- inch pieces)
- 1 cup coarsely chopped spinach
- 2 small Roma tomatoes, chopped

Directions:

1. Place the rack about 5-6 inches below the heating element in the oven. Set the oven to broil mode and preheat the oven.
2. Meanwhile, add eggs, milk, egg whites, and pepper into a bowl and whisk well.
3. Stir in chives and ¼ cup cheese.
4. Place a nonstick, ovenproof skillet over medium heat. Pour oil into the skillet and let it heat. When oil is hot, add green onion and asparagus and sauté for a couple of minutes.
5. Stir in garlic and cook for a few seconds until you get a nice aroma.
6. Stir in spinach and cook until spinach wilts. Spread the vegetables all over the skillet.
7. Drizzle the egg mixture all over the vegetables. Cook covered on low heat for about 10-12 minutes until the eggs are almost set. Scatter remaining cheese on top and shift the skillet into the oven. Broil for a couple of minutes until the cheese melts.
8. Scatter tomatoes on top.
9. Cut into four equal wedges and serve.

ENERGY BAR (SNACK)

Number of servings:	Nutritional values per serving:			
	Calories: 412	Carbohydrate: 36g		Protein: 12g
16	Fat: 26g	Fiber: 7g		

Ingredients:

- 2 cups roughly chopped almonds
- 1 cup honey or maple syrup
- 4 tablespoons melted coconut oil

- 3 cups uncooked quick cooking oats
- 2 cups almond butter or peanut butter
- 1 teaspoon salt (optional)

- 2 cups dried cranberries or chocolate chips or dried tart cherries or dried fruit or nuts

Directions:

1. Combine oats, almonds, and cranberries in a large bowl.
2. Combine coconut oil and almond butter in a small saucepan. Place the saucepan over low heat and cook the mixture until smooth.
3. Turn off the heat. Add honey and stir. Pour into the bowl of oat mixture and mix well.
4. Spread the mixture into a large baking dish. Press the mixture well onto the bottom of the dish.
5. Make marking for 16 equal size bars. Keep the dish covered in cling wrap and chill for 3-8 hours.
6. Now cut over the markings. Place in an airtight container in the refrigerator. It can last for 6-7 days in the refrigerator or for a month in the freezer.
7. Thaw before serving.

QUINOA AND BLACK BEAN SALAD (LUNCH)

	Nutritional values per serving: 1 ½ cups		
Number of servings: 3	**Calories:** 458 **Fat:** 26g	**Carbohydrate:** 46,5g **Fiber:** 9,6g	**Protein:** 13,8g

Ingredients:

- 1 ear corn, remove husk
- 3 tablespoons extra-virgin olive oil
- ¾ teaspoon ground cumin
- 1 ½ cups baby arugula
- ½ cup Pico de Gallo, divided
- 6 tablespoons cotija

- cheese, divided
- ½ medium zucchini, cut into ¼ inch thick slices lengthwise
- 2 tablespoons lime juice
- 1 ½ cups cooked quinoa
- ½ can (from a 15 ounces

- can) unsalted black beans, drained, rinsed
- ¼ cup chopped cilantro
- ½ avocado, peeled, pitted, diced, divided

Directions:

1. Follow the instructions on the package of quinoa and cook quinoa. Measure out 1 ½ cups of quinoa and add into a large bowl. Add black beans and toss well.
2. Set up your grill and preheat the grill to medium heat. You can also grill in a grill pan if desired. If using a grill pan, spray the pan with cooking spray and place it over medium-high heat. Choose the method of grilling.
3. Place zucchini on the grill and cook for about two minutes on each side. Take out the zucchini and place on your cutting board.
4. Grill the corn on all the sides until tender and cooked to your preference.
5. When corn is cool enough to handle, remove the corn kernels from the cob.
6. Chop the zucchini into smaller pieces. Add corn, zucchini, arugula, ¼ cup Pico de Gallo, 1/8 cup cilantro, half the avocado and three tablespoons cheese into the bowl of quinoa and toss well.
7. To make dressing: Combine lime juice, oil and cumin in a small bowl. Whisk well and pour over the salad. Toss well.
8. Garnish with remaining Pico de Gallo, cheese, cilantro, and avocado and serve.

GREEN VEGGIE BOWL WITH CHICKEN AND LEMON-TAHINI DRESSING (DINNER)

	Nutritional values per serving:			
	One chicken cutlet with one cup vegetables, ½ cup rice and two tablespoons dressing			
Number of servings:	**Calories:**	452	**Carbohydrate:**	41,8g	**Protein:**	34,9g
2	**Fat:**	17,6g	**Fiber:**	5,3g		

Ingredients:

- For lemon tahini dressing:
- 2 tablespoons tahini
- 2 tablespoons lemon juice
- 2 tablespoons cold water
- ¼ teaspoon minced garlic
- Kosher salt to taste
- A large pinch ground cumin

For chicken and vegetables:
- 1 tablespoon water

- 1 clove garlic, peeled, sliced
- Kosher salt to taste
- ½ small head broccoli, cut into florets (about ½ cup)
- 1/8 teaspoon black pepper
- ¼ large onion, sliced
- 1 cup cooked brown rice
- ½ cup trimmed, halved green beans

- 2 chicken cutlets (4 ounces each), trimmed
- 1 tablespoon extra-virgin olive oil, divided
- 2 cups thinly sliced kale
- 1/8 cup chopped fresh cilantro

Directions:

1. To make dressing: Combine all the dressing ingredients in a bowl. Whisk well. Cover and set it aside for a while for the flavors to blend.
2. Pour ½ tablespoon oil into a cast-iron skillet and place the skillet over medium heat.
3. Sprinkle salt and pepper over the chicken and place in the skillet. Cook for 3-5 minutes on each side.
4. The internal temperature of the chicken when checked with a meat thermometer should show 160°F on a meat thermometer.
5. Remove chicken from the pan and place on a plate. Cover the plate loosely with foil.
6. Clean the pan and add ½ tablespoon oil. Place the skillet over medium heat. When oil is hot, add onion and cook for a couple of minutes until it turns translucent.
7. Stir in garlic and cook for a few seconds until fragrant.
8. Stir the broccoli and green beans into the pan and cook for a couple of minutes.
9. Add kale and a tablespoon of water and cover the pan. Cook for a couple of minutes until the vegetables are bright green in color. They should be crisp as well as tender.
10. Cut the chicken into slices if desired.
11. To assemble: Take two bowls and place ½ cup rice in each bowl. Layer with half the vegetables in each bowl. Place a sliced chicken cutlet over the vegetables in each bowl.
12. Pour dressing on top. Garnish with cilantro and serve.

WEDNESDAY

APPLE PANCAKES (BREAKFAST)

Nutritional values per serving:
Two pancakes

Number of servings:	**Calories:**	346	**Carbohydrate:**	54g	**Protein:**	12g
6	**Fat:**	10g	**Fiber:**	8g		

Ingredients:

- 2 apples, peeled, cored, finely diced
- 2 cups oat milk
- 4 tablespoons maple syrup or honey
- ¼ teaspoon ground nutmeg

- 1 teaspoon baking powder
- 1 cup chopped mixed dried fruit and nuts
- 2 medium eggs
- 3 cups rolled oats or quick oats

- 4 teaspoons ground cinnamon
- ¼ teaspoon salt
- ¼ cup hemp seeds
- Olive oil cooking spray

Directions:

1. Blend together oat milk, honey, nutmeg, baking powder, nuts, eggs, oats, cinnamon and salt in a blender until smooth.
2. Pour into a bowl. Add hemp seeds and stir. Give the batter some rest for about 2-3 minutes.
3. Place a nonstick pan over medium heat. When the pan is hot, spray the pan with cooking spray.
4. Pour about ¼ cup of batter on the pan. Scatter a little of the apples over the batter (make 12 equal portions of the apple and scatter a portion of the apple).
5. Press the apples lightly into the batter to adhere. Cook until the underside is golden brown.
6. Turn the pancake over and cook the other side as well. Remove the pancake from the pan and keep warm.
7. Make the remaining pancakes similarly (Steps 3-6, make sure to spray the pan each time you make a pancake). You should have 12 pancakes in all.
8. Serve warm with a tablespoon of maple syrup for each serving, the nutritional value of which is not included.

SPICY CUCUMBER MINT SMOOTHIE (SNACK)

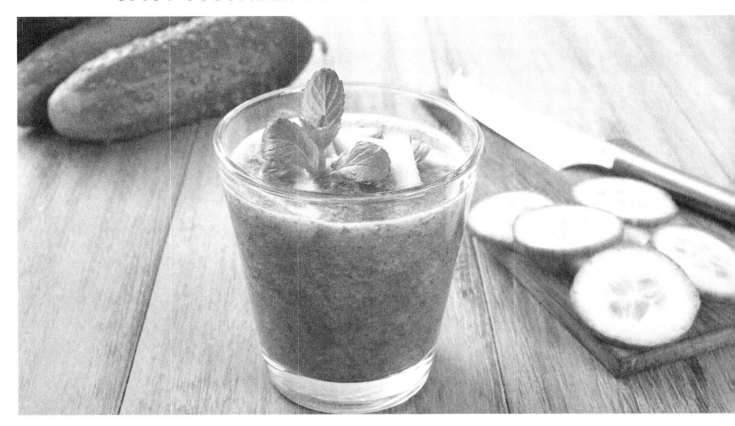

	Nutritional values per serving: One glass		
Number of servings: 2	**Calories:** 437 **Fat:** 35g	**Carbohydrate:** 20g **Fiber:** 10g	**Protein:** 18g

Ingredients:

- 1 teaspoon extra-virgin coconut oil
- 2 tablespoons raw almond butter
- ½ cup hemp seeds
- 1 small cucumber, peeled, chopped
- 2 kale leaves, discard hard stems and ribs, torn
- 4-6 ice cubes
- ½ jalapeño chili, deseeded, chopped (optional)
- 1 inch fresh ginger, peeled, sliced
- 2 tablespoons chia seeds
- ½ avocado, peeled, pitted, chopped
- Juice of ½ lime
- 2 cups filtered water
- A handful fresh mint leaves

Directions:

1. Add coconut oil, almond butter, hemp seeds, cucumber, kale, jalapeño, ginger, chia seeds, avocado, lime juice, water, and mint leaves into a blender and blend until you get a smooth texture.
2. Pour into two glasses and serve with ice.

CALIFORNIA STEAK SALAD (LUNCH)

	Nutritional values per serving:		
	Three ounces steak with 1 ½ cups salad		
Number of servings:	**Calories:** 280	**Carbohydrate:** 14g	**Protein:** 16g
2	**Fat:** 18,8g	**Fiber:** 5g	

Ingredients:

- ½ large red onion, cut into ½ inch thick wedges
- ½ tablespoon balsamic vinegar
- Freshly ground black pepper to taste
- 2.5 ounces arugula

- ½ ripe avocado, peeled, pitted, sliced
- 1/8 cup sliced, toasted almonds
- 1 tablespoon extra-virgin olive oil
- ¼ teaspoon kosher salt

- 1 ½ medium tomatoes, sliced
- 6 ounces cooked flank steak seasoned with salt and pepper
- ¼ cup thinly sliced basil

Directions:

1. Place a grill pan over high heat. Spray some cooking spray into the pan. When the pan is hot, add onion and cook until slightly charred. Turn the onions every 3-4 minutes.
2. Transfer the onion into a bowl. Cover the bowl with cling wrap. Let the onion rest for 10 minutes.
3. Add vinegar, oil, pepper, and salt into another bowl and whisk well. Add the onions into the bowl along with any of the released juices.
4. Stir in the tomatoes as well. Let it marinate for 15 minutes.
5. Add arugula and stir.
6. Divide the salad into two plates. Place steak and avocado on top.
7. Garnish with basil and almonds and serve.

GREEK PASTA (DINNER)

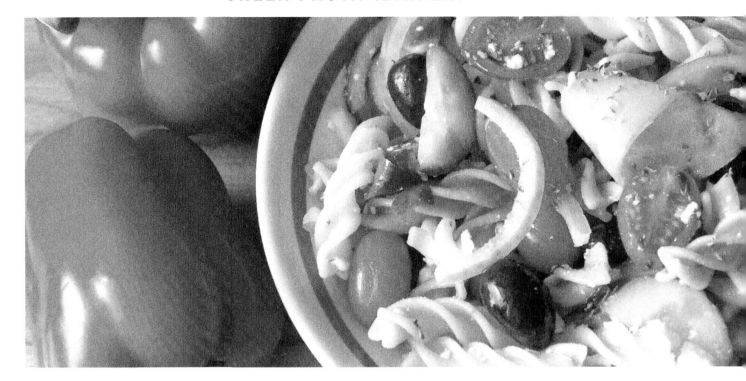

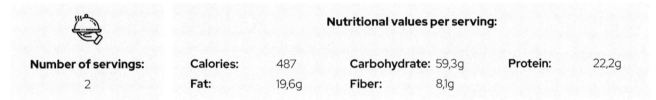

Nutritional values per serving:

Number of servings:	Calories:	487	Carbohydrate:	59,3g	Protein:	22,2g
2	Fat:	19,6g	Fiber:	8,1g		

Ingredients:

- 1 tablespoon olive oil
- ½ cup diced onion
- ½ can (from an eight ounces can) unsalted tomato sauce
- 3 cups cooked whole wheat rotini pasta
- ¼ cup finely crumbled feta cheese
- 4.5 ounces cooked chicken sausage, cut into round slices
- 2 small cloves garlic, peeled, minced
- 2 cups baby spinach
- 1/8 cup pitted, chopped kalamata olives
- 1/8 cup chopped fresh basil

Directions:

1. Place a skillet over medium- high heat. Add oil. When oil is hot, add sausage, garlic, and onion and cook until onion is light brown.
2. Stir in spinach, tomato sauce, olives, and pasta and toss well. Heat thoroughly. Cook until spinach wilts.
3. Sprinkle some water if the sauce is very thick.
4. Add feta cheese and basil and mix well.
5. Serve.

THURSDAY

BERRY CHIA PUDDING (BREAKFAST)

Nutritional values per serving:
One glass

Number of servings: 4	**Calories:** 343	**Carbohydrate:** 39,4g	**Protein:** 13,8g
	Fat: 15,4g	**Fiber:** 14,9g	

Ingredients:

- 3 ½ cups blackberries or raspberries or diced mangoes, divided
- ½ cup chia seeds
- 1 ½ teaspoons vanilla extract
- ½ cup granola
- 2 cups unsweetened almond milk or milk choice
- 2 tablespoons maple syrup
- 1 cup whole-milk plain Greek yogurt

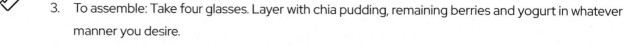

Directions:

1. Blend together 2 ½ cups berries and milk in a blender until very smooth.
2. Pour into a bowl. Add chia seeds, vanilla, and maple syrup and stir. Cover the bowl with cling wrap and chill overnight. This can last for three days.
3. To assemble: Take four glasses. Layer with chia pudding, remaining berries and yogurt in whatever manner you desire.
4. Top each glass with two tablespoons granola and serve.

PEACH TOAST WITH PISTACHIOS (SNACK)

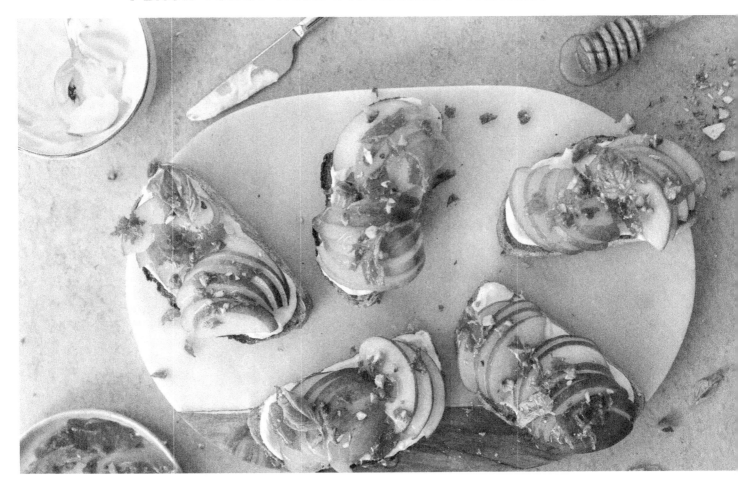

Nutritional values per serving:
One toast

Number of servings:	Calories:	193	Carbohydrate:	29g	Protein:	8,2g
2	Fat:	6g	Fiber:	3,9g		

Ingredients:

- 2 tablespoons part-skim ricotta cheese
- ½ teaspoon ground cinnamon
- 1 medium peach, pitted, sliced
- 2 teaspoons honey, divided
- 2 slices 100% whole wheat bread, toasted
- 2 tablespoons chopped pistachios

Directions:

1. Place ricotta, cinnamon and one teaspoon honey in a bowl and stir well.
2. Spread this mixture over the toasted bread slices. Place peach slices on top.
3. Scatter pistachios on top. Trickle ½ teaspoon honey on each toast and serve.

CHICKPEA AND QUINOA GRAIN BOWL (LUNCH)

		Nutritional values per serving: One bowl		
Number of servings: 2	**Calories:** **Fat:**	503 16,6g	**Carbohydrate:** 75g **Fiber:** 16,1g	**Protein:** 17,9g

Ingredients:

- 2 cups cooked quinoa
- 1 cup diced cucumber
- ½ avocado, peeled, pitted, diced
- 1/8 cup finely chopped roasted red pepper
- 1/8 cup water + more if required
- Salt to taste
- 2/3 cup cooked or canned chickpeas, rinsed, drained
- 1 cup halved cherry tomatoes
- 6 tablespoons hummus
- 2 tablespoons lemon juice
- 2 teaspoons finely chopped parsley
- Ground pepper to taste

Directions:

1. To make dressing: Whisk together hummus, water, lemon juice, red pepper, and lemon juice into a bowl. Add more water if the dressing is very thick.
2. Stir in parsley, salt, and pepper.
3. Take two bowls. Layer the bowls with equal quantities of quinoa followed by chickpeas and cucumber.
4. Next layer with tomatoes and finally avocado. Drizzle the dressing on top and serve.

TACO-STUFFED SWEET POTATOES (DINNER)

Nutritional values per serving:
½ stuffed sweet potato

Number of servings:	Calories:	510	Carbohydrate:	34,6g	Protein:	41,2g
2	Fat:	23g	Fiber:	6,4g		

Ingredients:

- 1 sweet potato (1 pound)
- ½ pound lean ground beef
- ½ tablespoon ground cumin
- ¼ teaspoon onion powder
- Salt to taste
- 1 tablespoon tomato paste
- ½ cup shredded romaine lettuce
- ½ tablespoon avocado oil
- ½ tablespoon chili powder
- ¼ teaspoon garlic powder
- 1/8 teaspoon ground
- chipotle chili
- 1/8 cup water
- ½ cup shredded Mexican cheese blend, divided
- 2 tablespoons Pico de Gallo

Directions:

1. Pierce the sweet potato at several places with a fork. Place in a microwave and cook until soft, about 10-12 minutes.
2. While the sweet potato is cooking, place a skillet over medium-high heat. Add oil. When oil is heated, add beef, salt, and spices and cook until meat is brown. While cooking, as you stir, break the meat into smaller pieces.
3. Combine water and tomato paste in a bowl and pour into the skillet. Mix well. Add ¼ cup cheese and stir.
4. Cut the sweet potato into two halves. Mash the center of sweet potato flesh a little using a fork.
5. Divide the beef mixture equally and place over the sweet potato halves. Top each half with half of each-cheese, lettuce and Pico de Gallo.

FRIDAY

CHOCOLATE CHIP OATMEAL COOKIE SMOOTHIE (BREAKFAST)

	Nutritional values per serving:				
Number of servings: 1	**Calories:** 320	**Fat:** 13,9g	**Carbohydrate:** 44,8g	**Fiber:** 7,7g	**Protein:** 9,3g

Ingredients:

- 2/3 cup unsweetened almond milk
- ½ tablespoon chia seeds
- 2 medjool dates, pitted, soaked in warm water for 20 minutes
- 1 tablespoon raw cacao nibs or dark chocolate chips
- ¼ teaspoon pure vanilla extract
- Ice cubes, as required
- ¼ cup rolled oats
- ½ small banana, sliced, frozen
- 1 tablespoon almond butter
- ½ teaspoon cocoa powder, unsweetened
- 3-4 drops almond extract

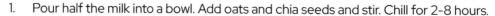

Directions:

1. Pour half the milk into a bowl. Add oats and chia seeds and stir. Chill for 2-8 hours.
2. Pour the mixture into a blender. Add remaining milk, dates, cocoa powder, vanilla, banana, almond butter, cacao nibs, and almond extract and blend until smooth.
3. Pour into a tall glass and serve.

GREEK CHEESE BALLS (SNACK)

Nutritional values per serving:

Number of servings:	Calories:	280	Carbohydrate:	5,3g	Protein:	15,6g
4	Fat:	34,1g	Fiber:	1g		

Ingredients:

- 4 ounces cream cheese, softened
- 1 tablespoon balsamic vinegar
- 4 ounces feta cheese, crumbled
- ½ tablespoon dried oregano
- ½ teaspoon garlic powder
- 6 tablespoons pine nuts, divided
- 4 tablespoons mayonnaise
- 5 ounces shredded cheddar cheese
- 1/8 cup grated Parmesan cheese
- 1 teaspoon onion powder
- 1/8 cup pecan halves

Directions:

1. Add cream cheese, vinegar, and mayonnaise into a bowl and stir until smooth.
2. Combine cheddar cheese, Parmesan cheese, feta cheese, garlic powder, onion powder, and oregano in another bowl and add it into the bowl of cream cheese.
3. Mix well. Divide the mixture into five equal portions and form into balls.
4. Place two tablespoons of pine nuts and pecans in the blender and give short pulses until crumb-like.
5. Transfer onto a plate. Add four tablespoons of pine nuts and stir until well combined.
6. Dredge the cheese balls in the pecan mixture. Press well the nut mixture on the cheese balls. Make sure the cheese ball is well coated.
7. Chill until use.

SPLIT PEA SOUP WITH BACON (LUNCH)

Nutritional values per serving:
1 1/3 cups

Number of servings:
4

Calories:	473	**Carbohydrate:**	59g	**Protein:**	26g
Fat:	11g	**Fiber:**	16g		

Ingredients:

- 3 ½ strips bacon
- 2 ½ medium stalks celery, sliced
- 4 cloves garlic, minced
- ¾ cup diced onion

- 1 ¾ cups cubed sweet potato
- 2 ½ teaspoons miso
- 3 ¼ cups chicken stock
- Pepper to taste

- ¾ teaspoon dried thyme
- Salt to taste
- 2 ½ cups water
- 12.8 ounces yellow or green split peas, rinsed well

Directions:

1. Place a heavy bottomed pot over medium heat. Add bacon and cook until brown around the edges.
2. Remove bacon with a slotted spoon and place on a plate lined with paper towels. When cool enough to handle, crumble the bacon.
3. Retain about a tablespoon of the bacon fat and discard the rest.
4. Add onion and celery into the pot and cook for a couple of minutes.
5. Stir in the sweet potatoes and allow it to cook for about two minutes.
6. Next add miso and garlic and cook for a few seconds until you get a nice aroma.
7. Add peas and mix well. Add broth and water and stir. Lower the heat and add thyme. Cover the pot partially and cook until the split peas are cooked until soft.
8. Add salt and pepper to taste.
9. Ladle into soup bowls. Sprinkle bacon on top and serve.

SALMON WITH ROASTED RED PEPPER QUINOA SALAD (DINNER)

Nutritional values per serving:

Number of servings:	**Calories:**	481	**Carbohydrate:** 31g	**Protein:**	35,8g
2	**Fat:**	21g	**Fiber:** 3,5g		

Ingredients:

- 1 ½ tablespoons extra-virgin olive oil, divided
- Salt to taste
- 1 tablespoon red wine vinegar
- 1 cup cooked quinoa

- 1/8 cup chopped fresh cilantro
- 10 ounces skin-on salmon, preferably wild caught, cut into two equal portions
- Pepper to taste

- 2 small cloves garlic, peeled, grated
- ½ cup chopped roasted red pepper (from jar), rinsed
- 1/8 cup toasted pistachios

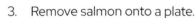

Directions:

1. Pour ½ tablespoon oil into a nonstick skillet. Place the skillet over medium-high heat.
2. Dry the salmon by patting it with paper towels. Season with salt and pepper and place in a pan with the skin side on top. Cook for 3-4 minutes. Turn the salmon over and cook for a couple of minutes or until cooked through.
3. Remove salmon onto a plate.
4. To make salad: Add one tablespoon oil, vinegar, salt, garlic, and pepper in a bowl and whisk well.
5. Stir in quinoa, cilantro, red pepper and pistachios.
6. Divide salad into two plates. Divide the salmon among the plates and serve.

S A T U R D A Y

BANANA, RAISIN, AND WALNUT BAKED OATMEAL (BREAKFAST)

Number of servings:	Nutritional values per serving:				
	Calories:	327	**Carbohydrate:** 46,2g	**Protein:**	9,1g
3	**Fat:**	13,1g	**Fiber:** 4,3g		

Ingredients:

- 1 cup rolled oats
- ¾ teaspoon ground cinnamon
- ¼ teaspoon salt
- 1 cup low-fat milk
- 1 tablespoon canola oil
- ½ teaspoon vanilla extract

- 3 tablespoons raisins
- 3 tablespoons chopped walnuts
- ½ teaspoon baking powder
- 1/8 teaspoon ground allspice
- 6 tablespoons low-fat plain

- yogurt
- 2 tablespoons packed light brown sugar
- ½ large banana, cut into half-moon slices

Directions:

1. You need to preheat your oven to 375°F. Grease a square baking dish of about (4-5 inches) with cooking spray.
2. Add oats, baking powder, salt, walnuts, and allspice in a bowl and stir.
3. Whisk together milk, oil, vanilla, yogurt, and brown sugar in another bowl. Once sugar dissolves, add raisins and banana slices and mix well.
4. Transfer the liquid mixture into the bowl of oats and mix well. Spoon the mixture into the prepared baking dish.
5. Place the baking dish in the oven and bake until golden brown on top.
6. Cut into three equal portions and serve.

PEANUT BUTTER COOKIE ENERGY BALLS (SNACK)

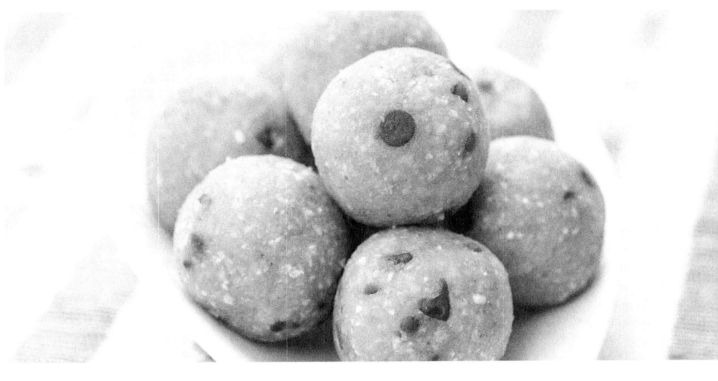

Nutritional values per serving:
One ball

Number of servings:	**Calories:** 318	**Carbohydrate:** 22g	**Protein:** 12g
5	**Fat:** 22,4g	**Fiber:** 5g	

Ingredients:

- ½ pound dry roasted unsalted peanuts
- ¼ teaspoon sea salt
- 2 tablespoons maple syrup
- 2 ounces pitted Deglet noor dates, quartered
- 1 tablespoon vanilla extract
- 1-2 tablespoons water

Directions:

1. Add dates and peanuts into the food processor bowl and process until chopped into smaller pieces.
2. Add vanilla, salt, and maple syrup and process until the mixture is sort of sticky when you press it together yet crumbly in texture.
3. Add a tablespoon of water and process until it sticks together. Add another tablespoon of water if required.
4. Once you get soft dough, transfer into a bowl.
5. Make five equal portions of the dough and shape into balls.
6. Transfer into an airtight container and refrigerate until use.

PAPRIKA CHICKEN THIGHS WITH BRUSSELS SPROUTS (LUNCH)

Nutritional values per serving:
One large or two small chicken thighs with ¾ cup vegetables

Number of servings:	Calories:	453	Carbohydrate:	14,3g	Protein:	44,1g
2	Fat:	24,6g	Fiber:	4,6g		

Ingredients:

- ½ pound Brussels sprouts, trimmed, halved or quartered depending on the size
- ½ lemon, cut into slices
- Salt to taste

- 1 clove garlic, minced
- ½ teaspoon dried thyme
- 2 small shallots, quartered
- 1 ½ tablespoons extra-virgin olive oil, divided
- Pepper to taste

- ½ tablespoon smoked paprika
- 2 large or four small chicken thighs, skinless

Directions:

1. Place the rack in the lower third position in the oven and preheat your oven to 450°F.
2. Place Brussels sprouts, lemon, and shallots in a bowl and toss well.
3. Drizzle a tablespoon of oil over the vegetables. Sprinkle salt and pepper and toss well.
4. Spread the mixture on a baking sheet.
5. Place garlic on your cutting board. Add a little salt and mash with a knife until you get a paste.
6. Add garlic, thyme, paprika, pepper, and ½ tablespoon oil into a bowl and mix well.
7. Rub this mixture all over the chicken. Place the chicken on the baking sheet as well.
8. Place the baking sheet in the oven and bake for about 20-30 minutes or until the internal temperature of the chicken in the thickest part of the meat shows 165°F on a meat thermometer.
9. Serve hot.

BROCCOLI QUINOA CASSEROLE (DINNER)

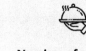

	Nutritional values per serving:			
	¼ of the recipe			
Number of servings:	**Calories:**	491	**Carbohydrate:** 61,3g	**Protein:** 27,6g
4	**Fat:**	16g	**Fiber:** 8,8g	

Ingredients:

- 2 cups quinoa, uncooked
- 1 ½ tablespoons pesto sauce
- 1 ½ teaspoons cornstarch or arrowroot powder
- 9.6 ounces fresh broccoli florets
- 1 3/3 cups fresh spinach
- 2 green onions, chopped
- 3 ¾ cups low sodium vegetable stock or water
- Pepper to taste
- ¼ cup shredded Parmesan cheese
- 9.6 ounces skim mozzarella cheese, shredded
- Salt to taste

Directions:

1. Grease a baking dish (9 x 13 inches) with some cooking spray. Set aside. Also preheat your oven to 400°F.
2. Cook broccoli in a microwave safe bowl, in a microwave for about three minutes or until it is crisp and as well as tender. Set aside.
3. Add stock, pesto, cornstarch, pepper, and salt into a bowl and whisk well.
4. Pour the mixture into a saucepan and place the saucepan over medium heat. Bring to a boil, stirring constantly.
5. Meanwhile, place quinoa, spinach Parmesan, most of the mozzarella cheese and green onions in the baking dish. Mix well. Pour the hot stock mixture over the quinoa.
6. Place the baking dish in the oven and bake for about 30 minutes.
7. Remove the dish from the oven. Add broccoli and stir well.
8. Sprinkle the rest of the mozzarella cheese over it. Bake for a few more minutes until the cheese melts.

SUNDAY

PEANUT BUTTER-BANANA CINNAMON TOAST (BREAKFAST)

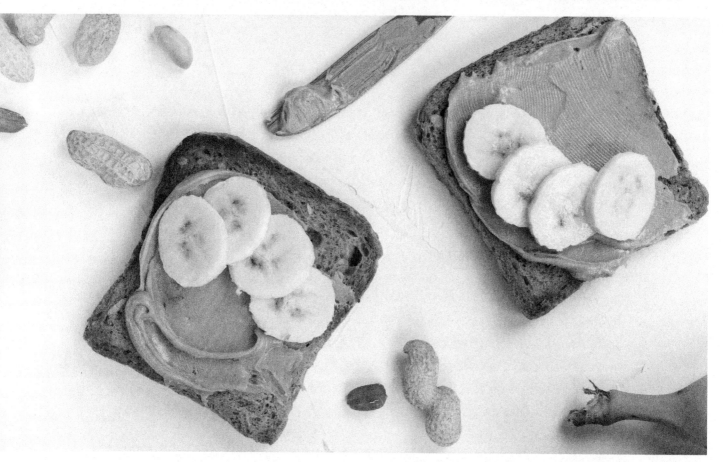

	Nutritional values per serving: Two toasts				
Number of servings: 1	**Calories:**	532	**Carbohydrate:** 76,6g	**Protein:**	16,2g
	Fat:	18,6g	**Fiber:** 11g		

Ingredients:

- 2 slices whole wheat bread
- 2 small bananas, sliced
- 2 tablespoons peanut butter
- Ground cinnamon to sprinkle

Directions:

1. Toast the bread slices to the desired doneness.
2. Spread a tablespoon of peanut butter on each toast. Place banana slices on top. Garnish with cinnamon and serve.

TOASTED BARLEY AND BERRY GRANOLA (SNACK)

Nutritional values per serving:
1/3 cup

Number of servings:	**Calories:**	181	**Carbohydrate:** 27,4g	**Protein:** 4,5g
6	**Fat:**	6,5g	**Fiber:** 3,7g	

Ingredients:

- 1/8 cup unsalted sunflower seed kernels
- 1/8 cup unsalted pumpkin seed kernels
- 3 tablespoons maple syrup
- 1 tablespoon canola oil
- ¾ teaspoon vanilla extract
- A pinch ground cardamom
- 1/8 cup toasted wheat germ
- 3 tablespoons sweetened dried cranberries
- 1 tablespoon brown sugar
- ½ teaspoon ground
- cinnamon
- 1/8 teaspoon salt
- 1 cup rolled barley flakes
- 3 tablespoons dried blueberries

Directions:

1. Set the temperature of your oven to 325°. Line a baking sheet with parchment paper.
2. Spread the pumpkin seeds and sunflower seeds on the baking sheet. Place the baking sheet in the oven and bake for five minutes.
3. Let it cool completely on your countertop.
4. Transfer the seeds into a bowl. Add barley flakes, salt, cinnamon, brown sugar, wheat germ, vanilla, oil, and maple syrup and mix well.
5. Spread the mixture on the baking sheet. Spread it evenly.
6. Bake the mixture until light brown. Make sure to stir the mixture every 8-10 minutes. Spread it all over the baking sheet each time you stir.
7. Cool completely. Transfer into an airtight container. Add blueberries and cranberries and mix well. Close the lid.
8. Store at room temperature.

MEDITERRANEAN VEGGIE WRAP (LUNCH)

	Nutritional values per serving:		
	One wrap		
Number of servings:	**Calories:** 239	**Carbohydrate:** 28g	**Protein:** 8g
4	**Fat:** 11g	**Fiber:** 6g	

Ingredients:

- 1 teaspoon olive oil
- 1 medium red bell pepper, thinly sliced
- 4 whole-grain wraps or tortillas
- 1 cup baby spinach leaves
- 2 teaspoons dried oregano
- 2 onions, thinly sliced
- 1 small zucchini, thinly sliced
- ½ cup hummus
- ¼ cup crumbled feta cheese
- 1/8 cup sliced black olives

Directions:

1. Pour oil into a skillet and place the skillet over medium-low heat. When oil is hot, add onion, zucchini, and bell pepper and cook until tender.
2. Heat the wraps following the instructions on the package.
3. Spread two tablespoons of hummus along the diameter of each wrap. Place ¼ cup spinach over the hummus.
4. Divide the vegetables equally and place over the spinach. Scatter oregano, olives, and feta cheese.
5. Wrap like a burrito. Cut each into two halves and serve.

BEEF AND VEGGIE BOWLS (DINNER)

	Nutritional values per serving:				
	One bowl				
Number of servings:	**Calories:**	556	**Carbohydrate:** 24g	**Protein:**	33g
2	**Fat:**	38g	**Fiber:** 8g		

Ingredients:

For beef:

- ½ pound lean ground beef
- ¼ teaspoon black pepper or to taste
- ¼ teaspoon salt or to taste
- ¼ teaspoon chili powder

For vegetables:

- 10-12 ounces fresh broccoli, cut into bite size florets
- ½ bell pepper, thinly sliced
- Salt to taste

- ¼ teaspoon garlic powder or to taste
- ½ pound Brussels sprouts, trimmed
- 1½ tablespoons extra-virgin olive oil
- ¼ teaspoon black pepper or to taste

For sauce:

- ¼ cup mayonnaise
- ½ teaspoon lemon juice
- ¼ teaspoon paprika
- ¼ teaspoon ground mustard
- ½ tablespoon ketchup
- ¼ teaspoon Tabasco or to taste
- ¼ teaspoon ground mustard

Directions:

1. To make sauce mixture: Combine all the ingredients for sauce in a bowl. Cover and set aside.
2. Set the temperature of your oven to 425°.
3. Place broccoli on one side of a baking sheet. Place Brussels sprouts next to the broccoli. Place bell peppers next to the Brussels sprouts. Make sure the vegetables are spread out well, without overlapping.
4. Trickle oil over the vegetables. Season with garlic powder, salt and pepper.
5. Place the baking sheet in the oven and roast the vegetables until they are cooked to your preference.
6. Meanwhile, place a skillet over medium-high heat. Add beef and cook until brown. As you stir, make sure to break the meat.
7. Add salt, pepper, and chili powder.
8. To assemble: Distribute the roasted vegetables equally into two bowls. Divide the meat among the bowls. Drizzle sauce on top and serve.

WEEK 2 - MONDAY

SRIRACHA, EGG AND AVOCADO OVERNIGHT OATS (BREAKFAST)

Nutritional values per serving:
One bowl

Number of servings:	**Calories:**	317	**Carbohydrate:** 34,9g	**Protein:**	12,7g
2	**Fat:**	15,2g	**Fiber:** 7,9g		

Ingredients:

- 1 cup rolled oats
- 1/8 cup chopped onion
- 4 cherry tomatoes, chopped
- 2 teaspoons sriracha
- 1 ½ cups water
- ½ avocado, peeled, pitted, sliced
- 2 large eggs, cooked sunny side up
- Salt to taste
- Pepper to taste

Directions:

1. Add oats and water into a microwave safe container. Cover the bowl and chill for 8-9 hours.
2. Add onion and stir. Place in the microwave and heat the mixture thoroughly.
3. Add salt and pepper to taste.
4. Divide the oats into two bowls. Scatter tomatoes and avocado on top. Place an egg on top, in each bowl. Sprinkle salt and pepper to taste.
5. Drizzle a teaspoon of sriracha in each bowl and serve.

ORANGE-HAZELNUT SNACK MUFFINS (SNACK)

Nutritional values per serving:
One muffin

Number of servings:	Calories:	81	Carbohydrate:	7,6g	Protein:	1,6g
6	Fat:	5g	Fiber:	0,5g		

Ingredients:

- ¾ ounce hazelnut flour
- ½ teaspoon baking powder
- 1 ¼ ounces cake flour
- 1/8 teaspoon salt
- 1 tablespoon 2% reduced-
- fat milk
- ¾ teaspoon grated orange rind
- 1 small egg, lightly beaten
- 1 tablespoon canola oil
- ¾ tablespoon agave nectar
- ½ tablespoon fresh orange juice

Directions:

1. Set the temperature of your oven to 350°F. Grease a six count mini muffin pan with some cooking spray. Place disposable liners as well.
2. Sift together cake flour, hazelnut flour, salt, and baking powder in a bowl.
3. Crack egg into another bowl. Add oil, agave nectar, orange juice, milk, and orange rind and whisk well.
4. Add the mixture of flour into the bowl of wet ingredients and stir until just combined, making sure not to over mix.
5. Pour the batter into the muffin cups. Make sure to divide the batter equally among the cups.
6. Place the muffin pan in the oven and bake for 12 minutes. To check if the muffins are done, insert a toothpick in the center of a muffin. Pull out the toothpick and check if any particles are stuck on the toothpick. If the toothpick is not clean, bake for another 2-5 minutes. If it's clean, turn off the oven and pull out the muffin pan.
7. Let the muffins cool for a few minutes on the pan itself. Take out the muffins from the pan and place on a wire rack to cool.
8. Serve. You can store the leftover muffins in an airtight container.

AVOCADO-SPINACH PANINI (LUNCH)

	Nutritional values per serving:		
Number of servings: 2	**Calories:** 390 **Fat:** 13g	**Carbohydrate:** 65g **Fiber:** 8g	**Protein:** 12g

Ingredients:

- 1 avocado, peeled, pitted, thinly sliced
- 1 tablespoon diced red onion
- 2 ciabatta rolls (4 ounces each), split
- ½ ounce smoked sun-dried tomatoes, julienned
- Salt to taste
- 1 cup lightly packed baby spinach
- Pepper to taste

Directions:

1. Divide equally the vegetables and sun-dried tomatoes and place on the bottom half of the ciabatta rolls.
2. Cover with the top halves of the rolls.
3. Grease the Panini maker with some cooking spray and preheat it. You can also make it in a grill pan. Place the sandwich in the Panini maker and grill for 3-4 minutes or until the way you prefer it cooked.
4. Remove the sandwich from the Panini maker and place on your cutting board. Cut into the desired shape and serve.
5. Cook the other sandwich in a similar manner.
6. Serve Panini with a side of sweet potato fries.

BAKED SWEET POTATO FRIES (SIDE DISH)

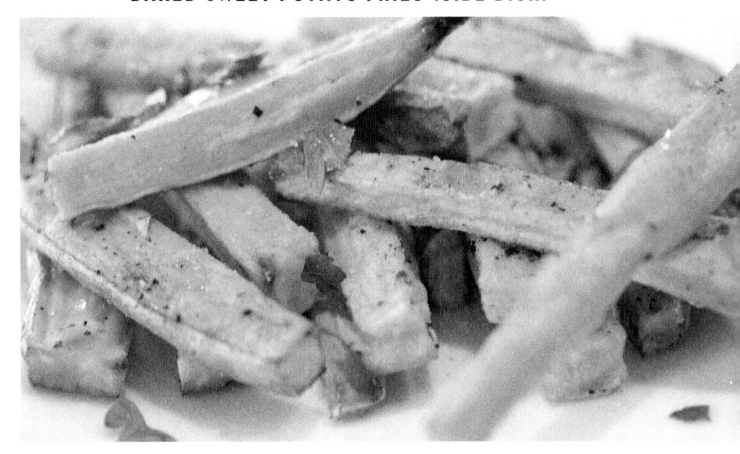

Nutritional values per serving:

Number of servings:	Calories:	236	Carbohydrate:	47,4g	Protein:	3,6g
2	Fat:	7,1g	Fiber:	6,8g		

Ingredients:

- 1 pound sweet potatoes, peeled, cut into fries
- ¼ teaspoon fine sea salt
- Spices of your choice
- ½ tablespoon cornstarch
- 1 tablespoon extra-virgin olive oil

Directions:

1. Set the temperature of your oven to 425°F. Line a baking sheet with parchment paper.
2. Place sweet potatoes on the baking sheet. Sprinkle cornstarch and toss well. Pour oil over them and toss once again. Spread it evenly all over the baking sheet without overlapping.
3. Place the baking sheet in the oven and bake until crisp. Stir every 5-6 minutes. Once they start getting brown, keep a watch over them as they can burn easily.
4. Transfer into a bowl. Sprinkle seasonings of your choice. Sprinkle salt and toss well.

LENTIL AND MUSHROOM STEW WITH POTATO PARSNIP MASH (DINNER)

	Nutritional values per serving:				
Number of servings: 2	**Calories:** 470	**Carbohydrate:** 66g	**Protein:** 15g		
	Fat: 16g	**Fiber:** 15g			

Ingredients:

For mash:
- ½ pound parsnip, peeled, chopped into chunks
- ½ pound Yukon gold or russet potatoes, partially peeled, chopped into chunks
- Salt to taste
- ¼ cup milk of your choice
- 1 tablespoon butter
- 1 teaspoon fresh rosemary

For stew:
- ½ yellow onion, finely chopped
- 4 ounces shiitake mushrooms, remove stem
- 1½ tablespoons tomato paste
- ½ tablespoon chopped fresh rosemary
- Salt to taste
- 1 cup vegetable broth
- ½ cup cooked brown lentils

- 1 tablespoon olive oil
- 4 ounces cremini mushrooms, sliced
- 2 cloves garlic, minced
- ¼ cup dry red wine
- 3 thyme sprigs
- ½ teaspoon black pepper or to taste
- 1 tablespoon flour
- 1 tablespoon soy sauce (optional)

Directions:

1. To make mash: Make sure the potatoes and parsnip are of the same size.
2. Cook potato and parsnip in a pot of water with a little salt added to it. When the vegetables are soft, turn off the heat and drain in a colander.
3. Transfer the vegetables into a bowl. Mash the mixture with a potato masher. Add butter, garlic, milk, and rosemary and mix well. Cover and keep warm.
4. While the potatoes and parsnip are cooking make the stew. Pour oil into a skillet and heat it over medium-high heat. When oil is hot, add onion and all the mushrooms and stir-fry until the mushrooms turn brown in color.
5. Stir in garlic and tomato paste and cook for about 3-4 minutes until the mixture turns sort of dark in color.
6. Pour wine and stir. Add rosemary, salt, thyme, and pepper and mix well. Let the wine reduce to half its original quantity.
7. Combine flour and broth in a bowl. Add soy sauce if using and whisk well. Add the stock mixture into the pan and mix well. Keep stirring until the stew is thick.
8. Add lentils and mix well. Heat thoroughly. Discard the thyme sprigs.
9. To assemble: Distribute equally the mash among two bowls. Divide the stew equally and pour over the mash.
10. Serve hot.

TUESDAY

CASSAVA FLOUR WAFFLES (BREAKFAST)

Number of servings:
1

Nutritional values per serving:
Without toppings

| Calories: | 724 | Carbohydrate: | 58g | Protein: | 11g |
| Fat: | 51g | Fiber: | 5g | | |

Ingredients:

- 1 egg
- ½ cup + 1/8 cup canned full-fat coconut milk (shake the can before pouring)
- 1 tablespoon butter, melted
- ½ cup cassava flour
- ½ teaspoon baking soda
- ½ teaspoon vanilla extract

Directions:

1. Crack egg into a bowl. Add coconut milk, butter, and vanilla and whisk well.
2. Add baking soda and flour and stir until just combined, making sure not to over mix but there should be no lumps in the batter.
3. Plug in your waffle maker and preheat it.
4. Spray the waffle maker with nonstick cooking spray.
5. Spoon the batter into the waffle maker. You should get a large waffle.
6. Follow the directions of the manufacturer's directions and cook the waffle until crisp.
7. Remove the waffle from the waffle maker and set it aside for a few minutes. It will crisp up a bit.
8. Serve.

GREEK YOGURT SPINACH ARTICHOKE DIP (SNACK)

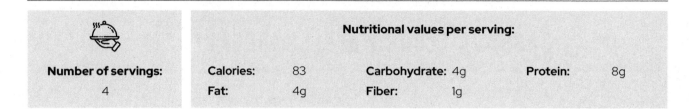

Number of servings:	Nutritional values per serving:		
	Calories: 83	**Carbohydrate:** 4g	**Protein:** 8g
4	**Fat:** 4g	**Fiber:** 1g	

Ingredients:

- 2.5 ounces frozen spinach, thawed
- ¼ can (from a 14 ounces can) artichoke hearts, drained, chopped
- 1.5 ounces feta cheese, crumbled
- 1 ½ tablespoons shredded Parmesan cheese + extra to top
- 3 tablespoons shredded mozzarella cheese + extra to top
- 3 tablespoons plain Greek yogurt
- ½ teaspoon minced garlic
- Serving options:
- Chips
- Crackers
- Vegetable sticks

Directions:

1. Set the temperature of the oven to 350°F and preheat the oven.
2. Prepare a small baking dish by greasing it with some cooking spray.
3. Squeeze the spinach of excess moisture.
4. Combine yogurt, spinach, feta, artichoke hearts, garlic, Parmesan, and mozzarella cheese in a bowl and spoon it into the baking dish.
5. Sprinkle some mozzarella cheese and Parmesan cheese on top.
6. Place the baking dish in the oven and bake until golden brown on top.
7. Serve with any of the serving options, the nutritional values of cheese topping and serving options is not mentioned. Adding it up will cover the calorie count of the day.

SEAFOOD COUSCOUS PAELLA (LUNCH)

	Nutritional values per serving:		
	1½ cups		
Number of servings:	**Calories:** 403	**Carbohydrate:** 60g	**Protein:** 27g
4	**Fat:** 7g	**Fiber:** 10g	

Ingredients:

- 4 teaspoons extra-virgin olive oil
- 2 cloves garlic, minced
- 1 teaspoon fennel seeds
- ½ teaspoon freshly ground pepper
- 2 cups unsalted, canned

- diced tomatoes, with juice
- 8 ounces small shrimp, peeled, deveined
- 8 ounces bay scallops, discard tough muscle
- 2 medium onion, chopped
- 1 teaspoon dried thyme

- ½ teaspoon salt or to taste
- A large pinch crumbled saffron threads
- ½ cup vegetable broth
- 1 cup whole-wheat couscous

Directions:

1. Place a large skillet or paella pan over medium heat. Add oil and let it heat. When oil is hot, add onion and sauté for a couple of minutes.
2. Stir in garlic, thyme, fennel seeds, salt, pepper, and saffron and sauté for a few seconds, until you get a nice aroma.
3. Add tomatoes and broth and mix well. When the mixture starts boiling, cook covered on low for 2-3 minutes.
4. Raise the heat to medium and add scallops. Stir occasionally and cook for 3-4 minutes. Stir in the shrimps and cook for another 2-3 minutes.
5. Add couscous and stir. Turn off the heat and keep the pan covered. Let it rest for about five minutes.
6. Fluff the paella with a fork.
7. Serve hot.

CHICKEN AND SPINACH SKILLET PASTA WITH LEMON AND PARMESAN (DINNER)

Number of servings:	Nutritional values per serving:				
2	Calories:	335	Carbohydrate:	24,9g	Protein: 28,7g
	Fat:	12,3g	Fiber:	2g	

Ingredients:

- 4 ounces gluten-free penne pasta or whole-wheat penne pasta
- ½ pound boneless, skinless chicken breast or thighs, trimmed, cut into bite size pieces
- Ground pepper to taste
- ¼ cup dry white wine
- 5 cups chopped fresh spinach
- 1 tablespoon extra-virgin olive oil
- ¼ teaspoon salt
- 2 cloves garlic, minced
- Juice of ½ lemon
- Zest of ½ lemon, grated
- 2 tablespoons grated Parmesan cheese, divided

Directions:

1. Follow the directions on the package of pasta and cook the pasta.
2. Place a skillet over medium-high heat. Pour oil and allow it to heat. When oil is hot, season chicken with salt and pepper and place in the pan. Cook until chicken is brown all over and cooked.
3. Stir in garlic and cook for a few seconds until you get a nice aroma. Add wine, lemon juice, and lemon zest and mix well.
4. When it starts simmering, turn off the heat. Add spinach and stir. Add pasta and toss well. Keep the pan covered for 5-8 minutes.
5. Distribute into two plates and serve.

WEDNESDAY

HONEY PECAN GRANOLA (BREAKFAST)

Nutritional values per serving:
One cup

Number of servings:	Calories:	677	Carbohydrate:	63,5g	Protein:	17,3g
2	Fat:	37,9g	Fiber:	12,8g		

Ingredients:

- 2.6 ounces rolled oats
- 0.9 ounce almonds
- 0.4 ounces pepitas
- 0.4 ounces sunflower seeds

- 1.8 ounces pecans
- ¼ teaspoon ground cinnamon
- 1 tablespoon extra-virgin olive oil

- Zest of ¼ orange, grated
- ½ tablespoon honey

Directions:

1. Set the temperature of your oven to 350°. Line a baking sheet with parchment paper.
2. Place all the ingredients in a bowl and toss well.
3. Spread the mixture on the baking sheet. Place the baking sheet in the oven and bake for eight minutes. Stir the mixture after four minutes of baking. Keep a watch over the granola as it can burn.
4. Let it cool completely on your countertop.
5. Transfer into an airtight container and store at room temperature.

COCONUT-DATE TRUFFLE BITES (SNACK)

Number of servings:
14

Nutritional values per serving:
One bite

Calories:	69	**Carbohydrate:**	9,1g	**Protein:**	1,2g
Fat:	4,1g	**Fiber:**	1,5g		

Ingredients:

- ½ cup roasted salted almonds
- ¼ cup flaked unsweetened coconut
- ½ tablespoon coconut oil
- 1 ounce bittersweet chocolate, chopped
- 15 whole dates, pitted
- 1 tablespoon unsweetened cocoa
- A pinch salt

Directions:

1. Grind the almonds in a food processor until finely powdered.
2. Place dates in the food processor and process until smooth.
3. Add oil, cocoa, salt, and coconut and give short pulses until just combined.
4. Make 14 equal portions of the mixture and shape into balls.
5. Place them on a plate lined with parchment paper. Chill for an hour.
6. Melt chocolate in a microwave. Dunk the truffles in chocolate, one at a time and place back on the plate.
7. Chill until the chocolate hardens.

GREEK KALE SALAD WITH QUINOA AND CHICKEN (LUNCH)

Number of servings:
1

Nutritional values per serving:

Calories:	301	**Carbohydrate:**	27,1g	**Protein:**	29,8g
Fat:	7,9g	**Fiber:**	3,7g		

Ingredients:

- 2 cups chopped kale
- ½ cup cooked quinoa
- ¼ cup Greek salad dressing
- ¾ cup cooked, shredded chicken
- 1/8 cup sliced roasted red pepper from jar
- ½ ounce crumbled feta cheese

Directions:

1. Combine chicken, kale, red pepper, and quinoa in a bowl. Pour dressing on top. Toss well.
2. Transfer into a bowl. Sprinkle feta on top and serve.

SHRIMP IN COCONUT SAUCE (DINNER)

	Nutritional values per serving:			
Number of servings:	**Calories:**	539	**Carbohydrate:** 10g	**Protein:** 38g
2	**Fat:**	39g	**Fiber:** 2g	

Ingredients:

- ¾ pound raw jumbo shrimp, peeled, deveined, remove shell and tail
- 2 small cloves garlic, minced
- 1 clove garlic, coarsely chopped
- Black pepper to taste
- ½ large red or orange bell pepper, sliced

- Few basil leaves , chopped and extra to garnish
- ½ cup canned coconut milk
- 1 tablespoon lime juice
- ½ teaspoon sweet paprika
- ½ red jalapeño pepper, thinly sliced (optional)
- 2 ½ tablespoons olive oil, divided
- Salt to taste

- 1 medium onion, chopped
- ¼ cup canned diced tomatoes
- 1 tablespoon chopped cilantro + extra to garnish
- 3 tablespoons chicken or vegetable broth
- ½ teaspoon ground ginger
- 3 ounces cream cheese, softened

Directions:

1. Combine shrimp, minced garlic, pepper, and salt in a bowl. Drizzle ½ tablespoon oil and toss well. Set it aside until the vegetables are cooked.
2. Pour one tablespoon of oil into a skillet and heat over medium heat. When oil is hot, add onion and bell pepper and sauté for a couple of minutes.
3. Stir in chopped garlic and cook for about a minute.
4. Stir in basil, tomatoes, and cilantro. Heat thoroughly. Transfer into a bowl and let it cool for a few minutes.
5. Pour one tablespoon of oil into the skillet. Add shrimp and cook for about two minutes on each side or until they turn pink. Remove shrimp onto a plate.
6. Place the tomato mixture into a blender. Add coconut milk, lime juice, broth, salt, ginger, paprika, and pepper and blend until smooth.
7. Pour the mixture into the skillet. Cook the mixture over medium heat. When it starts boiling, lower the heat and simmer for 3-4 minutes.
8. Stir in cream cheese. Stir often until cream cheese melts and the sauce is smooth.
9. Add shrimp and mix well. Transfer into a serving bowl.
10. Sprinkle cilantro, basil, and jalapeño slices on top.
11. You can serve it over cauliflower rice or zucchini noodles, the nutritional values are not included.

THURSDAY

OAT AND BERRY SMOOTHIE (BREAKFAST)

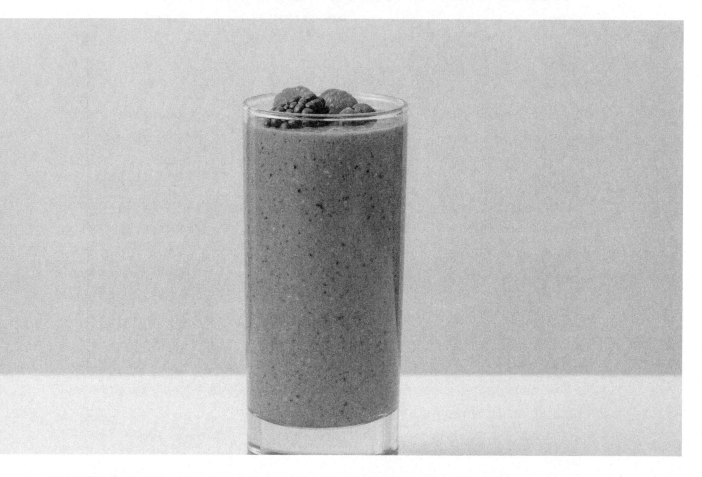

	Nutritional values per serving:		
Number of servings:	**Calories:** 295	**Carbohydrate:** 44g	**Protein:** 18g
1	**Fat:** 5g	**Fiber:** 7g	

Ingredients:

- ½ cup frozen berries of your choice
- 1/8 cup milk
- ¼ cup Greek yogurt
- 1 teaspoon honey
- 3 tablespoons oats

Directions:

1. Add berries, milk, yogurt, honey and oats into a blender.
2. Blend until you get a smooth texture.
3. Pour into a glass and serve.

GRILLED SHRIMP AND CUCUMBER GAZPACHO (SNACK)

Nutritional values per serving:
One cup soup with about 10 shrimp

Number of servings:	Calories:	318	Carbohydrate:	13g	Protein:	33g
2	Fat:	19g	Fiber:	3g		

Ingredients:

- 2 tablespoons sesame seeds, toasted
- ¼ sweet onion, chopped
- 1/8 cup Italian parsley
- 2 tablespoons olive oil, divided
- ½ tablespoon sherry vinegar or white wine vinegar

- ¼ teaspoon white pepper
- ½ teaspoon smoked paprika
- 1 cucumber, deseeded, chopped
- ½ clove garlic, peeled
- 1 ounce soft silken tofu
- 1 ½ tablespoons lime juice
- Salt to taste

- ½ pound shrimp, peeled, deveined (about 20 shrimp)
- White pepper to taste
- Bamboo skewers soaked in water for about 30 minutes (optional)

Directions:

1. This soup can be made a day in advance. Blend together cucumber, garlic, tofu, lime juice, onion, parsley, 1 ½ tablespoons oil, and vinegar in a blender until very smooth.
2. Pour into a container. Add salt and pepper to taste and mix well. Cover the container and chill until ready to serve.
3. You can grill the shrimp in a grill pan or on a preheated grill.
4. Drizzle ½ tablespoon oil over the shrimp. Add salt and paprika and toss well.
5. Grill the shrimp in the chosen method until they turn pink and hazy. It should take about three minutes on each side.
6. Divide the soup equally into two soup bowls. Top with shrimp. Sprinkle sesame seeds on top and serve.

NIÇOISE SALAD (LUNCH)

	Nutritional values per serving:		
Number of servings: 3	**Calories:** 435 **Fat:** 30g	**Carbohydrate:** 26g **Fiber:** 8,3g	**Protein:** 20g

Ingredients:

- 2 large eggs, hardboiled, peeled, halved
- 6 ounces haricot verts or green beans
- ½ tablespoons capers, drained, dried with paper towels
- 1 teaspoon Dijon mustard
- ½ teaspoon flaky sea salt
- 4 ounces bonito tuna
- packed in olive oil, divided
- 1 avocado, peeled, pitted, quartered
- ¼ cup pickled radishes
- ½ pound baby purple or red potatoes, halved if they are large
- 2 ½ tablespoons extra-virgin olive oil, divided
- 1 tablespoon red wine
- vinegar
- 1 tablespoon finely chopped dill + extra to garnish
- 1 ½ cups mixed greens
- 4 ounces grape tomatoes, halved
- 2 ounces nicoise olives

Directions:

1. Boil a pot of water. Add potatoes and cook until fork tender.
2. Now add haricot verts into the pot and cook for a couple of minutes. Drain the vegetables in a colander. Pick out the potatoes and place in a bowl.
3. Place the halved eggs on a serving platter.
4. Place a small pan over medium heat. Add one tablespoon of oil and let it heat. Add capers into the pan and move a bit away from your stove top as the capers can explode. After about a minute, turn off the heat and stir.
5. Pour the capers and oil over the eggs.
6. Combine 1 ½ tablespoons oil, mustard, salt, and dill in a small bowl. Drizzle a tablespoon of the dressing over the potatoes. Toss well and place the potatoes next to the eggs.
7. Place greens next to the potatoes followed by haricot verts and tuna. Next place tomatoes and avocado followed by olives and finally pickled radish.
8. Drizzle remaining dressing over the salad.
9. Sprinkle dill on top and serve.

TEMPEH BUDDHA BOWL (DINNER)

	Nutritional values per serving:			
Number of servings:	**Calories:**	523	**Carbohydrate:** 64,9g	**Protein:** 25,7g
2	**Fat:**	21,3g	**Fiber:** 14,7g	

Ingredients:

For marinating tempeh:

- 4 ounces tempeh, cubed
- ½ tablespoon maple syrup or agave
- ½ tablespoon rice wine vinegar
- Pepper to taste
- 1 tablespoon almond butter or any nut butter of your choice
- 1 ½ tablespoons tamari or soy sauce
- ½ teaspoon garlic powder

For dressing:

- 2 ½ tablespoons tahini
- ½ tablespoon rice wine vinegar
- 2 teaspoons tamari or soy sauce
- 1-2 tablespoons water

For the bowls:

- 1 cup cooked edamame
- ½ cup finely shredded red cabbage
- 2 cups chopped kale leaves
- 1 cup cooked brown rice
- ½ cup cooked corn kernels
- 2 medium onion, grated or julienned

Directions:

1. Combine maple syrup, vinegar, pepper, almond butter, tamari, and garlic powder in a bowl. Make sure the marinade is whisked until smooth.
2. Place tempeh in the bowl. Stir until tempeh is well coated with the marinade. Cover the bowl and chill for 1-2 hours.
3. Set the temperature of your oven to 375°F and preheat the oven. Prepare a baking sheet by lining it with parchment paper.
4. Remove tempeh from the bowl and place on the baking sheet.
5. Place the baking sheet in the oven and bake for 20 minutes.
6. Meanwhile, make the dressing: Whisk together tahini, vinegar, soy sauce and water in a bowl. If the dressing is very thick, add more water, a teaspoon at a time and whisk well each time.
7. Place kale in a skillet and place the skillet over medium heat. Sprinkle some water over the kale and cook until the kale wilts.
8. To assemble: Divide equally the edamame, cabbage, kale, brown rice, corn, onion, and tempeh into two bowls.
9. Divide the dressing among the bowls and serve.

FRIDAY

COCONUT MILK CHIA PUDDING (BREAKFAST)

Number of servings:

1

Nutritional values per serving:

Calories:	607	**Carbohydrate:**	48g	**Protein:**	7,8g
Fat:	46g	**Fiber:**	11g		

Ingredients:

- ½ cup coconut milk
- 2 tablespoons chia seeds
- 1 teaspoon vanilla extract
- 2 tablespoons coconut cream
- 2 tablespoons shredded coconut
- ½ tablespoon maple syrup
- For topping:
- 4-5 blueberries
- 4-5 raspberries
- 1 teaspoon shredded coconut, unsweetened

Directions:

1. Combine coconut milk, chia seeds, vanilla extract, coconut cream, shredded coconut, and maple syrup in a serving bowl.
2. Keep the bowl covered in the refrigerator overnight.
3. Scatter berries and shredded coconut on top and serve.

ROASTED RED PEPPER AND TOMATO SOUP (SNACK)

Nutritional values per serving:

Number of servings:			
3			

| Calories: | 170 | Carbohydrate: 14,2g | Protein: | 7,6g |
| Fat: | 5,9g | Fiber: | 3,5g |

Ingredients:

- ½ teaspoon olive oil + extra to brush
- 1 clove garlic, minced
- 2 large tomatoes, peeled, deseeded, chopped
- 1 teaspoon paprika or to taste
- 3 cups chicken broth
- A pinch cayenne pepper powder
- 1 tablespoon butter, melted
- 3 tablespoons sour cream
- ½ onion, chopped
- 1½ red bell peppers,
- ¾ teaspoon dried thyme
- Pepper to taste
- A pinch sugar
- Salt to taste
- Hot pepper sauce to taste
- ¾ tablespoon all-purpose flour or whole-wheat flour

Directions:

1. Set up your oven to broil mode and preheat the oven.
2. Brush oil on the bell pepper and place on the rack in the oven. Broil until charred. Turn the peppers each time a side gets charred.
3. Remove the bell peppers from the oven and place in a paper bag. Seal the bag and set it aside for 15 minutes. Peel the skin and chop the pepper.
4. Add oil into a pan over medium heat. When oil is hot, add garlic and onion and cook until onion turns pink.
5. Retain a little of the chopped peppers and add the rest into the pan. Also add tomatoes, sugar, paprika, and thyme and mix well.
6. Lower the heat to medium-low heat and cook until nearly dry.
7. Add stock, hot sauce, and seasonings and bring to a boil.
8. Now lower the heat and cover the pan partially. Cook until vegetables are soft.
9. Turn off the heat and let the soup cool for a while. Transfer the soup into a blender and blend until smooth.
10. Pour the soup into the pan. Combine butter and flour in a bowl and pour into the pan. Stir until the soup thickens. Stir in the retained red peppers.
11. Simmer for about five minutes on low heat.
12. Divide the soup equally among three bowls and serve garnished with sour cream.

STEAK SALAD WITH LETTUCE AND TOMATOES (LUNCH)

	Nutritional values per serving:		
Number of servings: 2	**Calories:** 370 **Fat:** 23g	**Carbohydrate:** 5g **Fiber:** 2g	**Protein:** 35g

Ingredients:

For vinaigrette:

- ½ tablespoon red wine vinegar
- ½ teaspoon Dijon mustard
- Pepper to taste
- ½ clove garlic, minced
- Kosher salt to taste
- 1 ½ tablespoons extra-virgin olive oil

For salad:

- ¼ cup halved cherry tomatoes
- 2 cups mixed salad greens

For steak:

- ½ teaspoon kosher salt
- ½ tablespoon paprika
- ½ teaspoon onion powder
- ¼ teaspoon pepper
- ½ teaspoon garlic powder
- ¼ teaspoon dried thyme
- ½ pound sirloin, cut into two inch cubes

Directions:

1. To make vinaigrette: Add vinegar, mustard, garlic, pepper, and salt in a bowl and whisk well.
2. Whisking constantly, pour oil in a thin drizzle. Keep whisking until emulsified. Cover and keep it aside for the flavors to meld.
3. Scatter mixed greens on a serving platter. Scatter tomatoes over the greens. Cover and keep it aside.
4. For steak: Combine salt and spices in a bowl. Add steak and mix well.
5. Pour oil into a skillet and heat it over medium-high heat. When oil is hot, add steak and cook to the desired doneness.
6. Scatter the steak over the salad. Give the vinaigrette a good stir. Spoon the vinaigrette over the salad and serve.

PAPRIKA CHICKEN THIGHS WITH BRUSSELS SPROUTS (DINNER)

Nutritional values per serving:
One large chicken thigh or two small chicken thighs with ¾ cup vegetables

Number of servings:	**Calories:**	453	**Carbohydrate:**	14,3g	**Protein:**	44,1g
2	**Fat:**	24,6g	**Fiber:**	4,6g		

Ingredients:

- ½ pound Brussels sprouts, trimmed, halved or quartered depending on the size
- ½ lemon, cut into slices
- Salt to taste

- 1 clove garlic, peeled, minced
- ½ teaspoon dried thyme
- 2 small shallots, quartered
- 2 large or four small, bone-in, skinless chicken thighs

- 1 ½ tablespoons extra-virgin olive oil, divided
- Pepper to taste
- ½ tablespoon smoked paprika

Directions:

1. Place the rack in the lower third position in the oven. Set the temperature of your oven to 450°F and preheat the oven.
2. Place Brussels sprouts, lemon slices, and shallots in a bowl. Add salt and pepper to taste. Drizzle a tablespoon of oil and toss well.
3. Spread the vegetables on a baking sheet. Mash garlic with a pinch of salt in a small bowl.
4. Add ½ tablespoon oil, paprika, pepper, and thyme and stir. Rub this mixture over the chicken. Place chicken on the baking sheet, along with the Brussels sprouts.
5. Place the baking sheet in the oven and roast until the chicken is cooked through and the internal temperature of the meat in its thickest part shows 165°F on a meat thermometer.

SATURDAY

MEDITERRANEAN BREAKFAST BURRITO (BREAKFAST)

Nutritional values per serving:
One burrito, without serving options

Number of servings: 3	**Calories:** 252	**Carbohydrate:** 21g
	Fat: 11g	**Fiber:** 2g

Protein: 14g

Ingredients:

- 3 whole-wheat tortillas (10 inches each)
- 1 cup baby spinach, rinsed, dried with paper towels
- 1½ tablespoons chopped sun-dried tomatoes
- 6 tablespoons canned refried beans
- 4 medium eggs
- 1½ tablespoons sliced black olives
- ¼ cup crumbled feta cheese
- Salsa and fruit to serve (optional)

Directions:

1. Place a skillet over medium heat. Spray some cooking spray.
2. Add eggs and stir frequently and cook until slightly soft.
3. Stir in spinach, sun-dried tomatoes and olives and cook until the eggs are well cooked.
4. Stir in feta cheese. Cover and cook for a minute or so until the cheese melts. Turn off the heat.
5. Spread tortillas on your countertop. Spread two tablespoons of refried beans on each tortilla.
6. Divide the spinach and egg mixture among the tortillas.
7. Fold one end of the tortilla such that the end touches the diameter of the tortilla. Fold once more and you will reach the other end of the tortilla. Repeat with all the tortillas.
8. Place the tortillas in a preheated Panini press and cook to the desired crispiness. You can also fry it in a skillet by spraying a bit of cooking spray.
9. Cut each into two halves and serve.

GREEK YOGURT SMOOTHIE WITH STRAWBERRIES (SNACK)

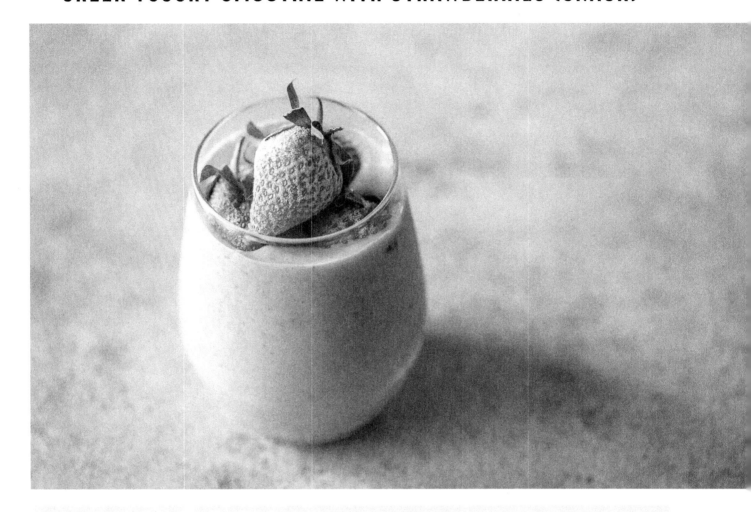

Number of servings:
2

Nutritional values per serving:

Calories: 392	**Carbohydrate:** 57g	**Protein:** 25g
Fat: 10g	**Fiber:** 7g	

Ingredients:

- 2 cups frozen strawberries
- 1 ½ cups plain, nonfat Greek yogurt
- 2 tablespoons peanut butter or almond butter
- Unsweetened almond milk or water, as required
- 2 medium bananas, sliced
- 4 tablespoons oatmeal
- Honey to taste (optional)

Directions:

1. Add strawberries, peanut butter, almond milk, yogurt, honey and oats into a blender.
2. Blend until you get a smooth texture.
3. Pour into two tall glasses and serve with crushed ice.

ROASTED MEDITERRANEAN VEGETABLE PASTA (LUNCH)

Nutritional values per serving:

Number of servings:			
2	Calories: 464	Carbohydrate: 62,2g	Protein: 15,3g
	Fat: 17,5g	Fiber: 12,6g	

Ingredients:

- 1 eggplant, cut into one inch cubes
- 1 yellow bell pepper, cut into one inch squares
- 1 zucchini (courgette), cut into one inch cubes
- ½ red onion, cut into one inch cubes
- 2 cloves garlic, peeled, crushed
- 12 cherry tomatoes
- 5.3 ounces whole-wheat pasta
- 10 basil leaves, torn
- 2 tablespoons olive oil
- 1 red chili pepper, sliced

Directions:

1. Set the temperature of your oven to 375°F and preheat the oven.
2. Place zucchini, eggplant, bell pepper, and onion in a baking dish.
3. Pour oil over the vegetables. Toss well and spread it evenly.
4. Place the baking dish in the oven and set the timer for 20 minutes or until the vegetables are cooked.
5. Follow the directions on the package of pasta and cook the pasta.
6. Transfer the drained pasta into a bowl. Add roasted vegetables and toss well.
7. Serve.

GRILLED FLANK STEAK AND CORN WITH GREEN GODDESS BUTTER (DINNER)

Nutritional values per serving:

Number of servings:		
2		

| Calories: | 420 | Carbohydrate: 20,3g | Protein: | 28,3g |
| Fat: | 26,3g | Fiber: | 2,3g | |

Ingredients:

- 2 tablespoons unsalted butter, softened
- 1 tablespoon chopped fresh chives
- ½ tablespoon fresh lemon juice
- ½ teaspoon salt, divided
- ½ pound flank steak, trimmed
- 2 ears corn, husked
- 1 tablespoon finely minced fresh basil
- 1 tablespoon finely minced fresh parsley + extra to serve
- ½ teaspoon chopped fresh thyme
- Pepper to taste
- ½ tablespoon extra-virgin olive oil
- 1/8 cup crumbled feta cheese

Directions:

1. Set up your grill and preheat it to medium-high heat.
2. To make green goddess butter: Combine butter, salt, pepper, lemon juice, and herbs in a bowl.
3. Cover the bowl and keep it aside.
4. Brush oil all over the steak and season with salt and pepper.
5. Place steak on the preheated grill and grill on both the sides until it is cooked as per your desire, medium-rare or rare or fully cooked.
6. Remove steak from the grill and place on your cutting board. Give it some rest for about 10 minutes.
7. Take about ½ tablespoon of the herb butter and spread it over the steak.
8. Once you take out the steak from the grill, place the corn on the grill and cook until a bit charred.
9. Remove corn and place it on your cutting board. Take the remaining herb butter and spread it on the corn.
10. Cut the steak into thin slices against the grain. Sprinkle salt to taste.
11. To serve: Divide steak slices into two serving plates. Place corn on each plate. Garnish with feta and parsley and serve.

S U N D A Y

GREEK YOGURT BREAKFAST BOWLS (BREAKFAST)

	Nutritional values per serving: One bowl				
Number of servings: 2	**Calories:** **Fat:**	267 2g	**Carbohydrate:** **Fiber:**	43g 6g	**Protein:** 21g

Ingredients:

- 1 ½ cups nonfat plain Greek yogurt
- 2 cups apples
- ½ teaspoon ground cinnamon
- 1 tablespoon maple syrup
- of honey
- ½ cup granola

Directions:

1. Divide yogurt into two serving bowls. Add ½ tablespoon maple syrup into each bowl and stir.
2. Divide the apples among the bowls. Top with ¼ cup granola in each bowl and serve.

APPLE PIE ENERGY BITES (SNACK)

		Nutritional values per serving: Two bites			
Number of servings: 3	**Calories:**	317	**Carbohydrate:** 38,9g	**Protein:**	9g
	Fat:	15g	**Fiber:** 7,6g		

Ingredients:

- 1 cup old fashioned rolled oats
- 1 tablespoon ground flaxseeds
- ½ tablespoon chopped hazelnuts
- ¼ teaspoon ground allspice

- ½ teaspoon vanilla extract
- 1/8 cup dried cranberries
- ½ teaspoon ground cinnamon
- ¼ teaspoon salt
- ½ tablespoon chopped walnuts

- ¼ cup almond butter
- 1 tablespoon honey
- ½ cup grated Granny Smith apples
- ½ teaspoon lemon juice

Directions:

1. As soon as you grate the apple, mix it up with lemon juice.
2. Combine oats, nuts, salt, and spices in a bowl.
3. Add almond butter into a microwave safe bowl and place it in the microwave for a few seconds until it melts a bit.
4. Add honey and vanilla and stir until well combined.
5. Add oat mixture and stir until well incorporated. Next add the apples and cranberries and stir well.
6. Make six equal portions of the mixture and shape into balls.
7. Place them on a plate. Chill for a while until firm. It can last for four days.

CAULIFLOWER RICE-STUFFED PEPPERS (LUNCH)

	Nutritional values per serving: One stuffed pepper					
Number of servings: 2	**Calories:**	374	**Carbohydrate:**	16,5g	**Protein:**	29,3g
	Fat:	21,7g	**Fiber:**	3,5g		

Ingredients:

- 2 large bell peppers of any color
- ¼ cup chopped onion
- 1 heaping cup cauliflower rice
- ½ pound lean ground beef
- 1 tablespoon extra-virgin olive oil, divided
- Pepper to taste
- ¼ teaspoon dried oregano
- Salt to taste
- ¼ cup shredded part-skim mozzarella cheese
- ½ can (from an eight ounces can) unsalted tomato sauce

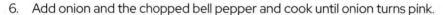

Directions:

1. Set the temperature of your oven to 375°F and preheat the oven.
2. Cut off a round slice of the bell pepper, near the stem. Do this with both the bell peppers. Now chop the part of the bell pepper from the cut slices. You should have around ½ cup of the chopped bell peppers.
3. Deseed the bell pepper and remove the membranes. Set the peppers aside.
4. Pour ½ tablespoon oil into a skillet and heat it over medium heat. When oil is hot, add cauliflower, a bit of salt and pepper and stir-fry until slightly brown and tender.
5. Spoon the cauliflower into a bowl. Clean the pan with a paper towel and pour remaining oil into the pan.
6. Add onion and the chopped bell pepper and cook until onion turns pink.
7. Add beef, garlic, oregano, pepper, and salt and mix well. Cook until the beef is not pink anymore. As you stir the mixture, break the meat into smaller pieces.
8. Stir in tomato sauce and cauliflower.
9. Turn off the heat.
10. Fill the mixture into the bell peppers. Place the bell peppers in a baking dish. Sprinkle cheese on top.
11. Bake the bell peppers for about 20–30 minutes until bell peppers are slightly tender and cheese melts.

BBQ RANCH CHICKEN QUINOA BOWLS (DINNER)

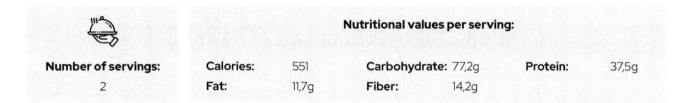

Nutritional values per serving:

Number of servings: 2	**Calories:** 551	**Carbohydrate:** 77,2g	**Protein:** 37,5g	
	Fat: 11,7g	**Fiber:** 14,2g		

Ingredients:

For chicken:
- ½ cup low-sugar BBQ sauce
- ½ pound boneless, skinless chicken breast
- 2 tablespoons water (only to be added if the sauce is thick)

For quinoa:
- 1 cup water
- ½ cup quinoa

For the bowls:
- ½ can (from a 15 ounces can) black beans
- ½ cup sweet corn, fresh or frozen
- 1 Roma tomato, diced
- ½ avocado, peeled, pitted, diced
- 1 cup shredded red cabbage
- 1/8 cup finely diced red onion
- ½ jalapeño, thinly sliced
- 4-5 tablespoons healthy Greek yogurt ranch dressing
- Sliced scallions to garnish
- Chopped cilantro to garnish

Directions:

1. If you have a slow cooker, cook the chicken in BBQ sauce in a slow cooker on High for 1 ½-2 hours, adding a little water if necessary.
2. If you do not have a slow cooker, cook it on the grill.
3. To cook on a grill: Combine chicken and BBQ sauce in a bowl and let it marinate for an hour.
4. Set up your grill and preheat it. Take out the chicken from the bowl and place it on the grill. Cook for 6-8 minutes on each side or until the internal temperature of the chicken in the thickest part of the meat shows 165°F on the meat thermometer.
5. Once cooked, shred the chicken with a pair of forks or chop into pieces and add it back into the pot/bowl. Mix well and keep warm until ready to eat.
6. To assemble: Take two serving bowls and divide the quinoa among the bowls. Divide equally the beans, cabbage, corn, onion, tomato, jalapeño, and avocado among the bowls. Place chicken over the vegetables.
7. Pour dressing on top. Sprinkle scallions and cilantro on top and serve.

WEEK 3 – MONDAY

CRUNCHY CORN WAFFLES (BREAKFAST)

Nutritional values per serving:

Calories:	300	**Carbohydrate:** 46g	**Protein:**	6g
Fat:	10g	**Fiber:**	8g	

Number of servings:
3

Ingredients:

- ½ cup + 1/8 cup unsweetened, plain non-dairy milk of your choice
- ¾ teaspoon cornstarch
- ½ teaspoon smoked sea salt or fine sea salt
- 2 tablespoons olive oil
- ½ cup whole wheat pastry

- flour or all-purpose flour
- 1 tablespoon nutritional yeast
- ¼ teaspoon baking soda
- ½ tablespoon apple cider vinegar
- 2 tablespoons water
- 1 tablespoon light brown

- sugar or sucanat
- 2 tablespoons fresh orange juice
- ½ cup medium-grind cornmeal
- 1 teaspoon baking powder
- ¼ teaspoon chipotle chili powder

Directions:

1. To make vegan buttermilk: Add non-dairy milk and vinegar into a cup. Stir it well and let it sit for 10-15 minutes. It will curdle.

2. Whisk together cornstarch and water in a heavy bottomed saucepan. Place the saucepan over medium heat and stir constantly until it turns thick, like jelly and sort of hazy in color. It should take no longer than 1½-2 minutes. Make sure you do not overcook else it will turn too thick and clump together.

3. Transfer the cornstarch mixture into the bowl of buttermilk. Whisk well. Add orange juice, water, oil, and sweetener and whisk well.

4. Add baking powder, chipotle chili powder, cornmeal, baking soda, and nutritional yeast into a bowl and stir. Add into the bowl of buttermilk mixture. Whisk until well combined. Set aside for at least 15 minutes.

5. Meanwhile, set up the waffle iron and preheat it following the manufacturer's instructions

6. Spray a generous amount of cooking spray in the waffle iron.

7. Pour 1/3 of the batter all over the waffle iron. When the waffle turns crisp (it should take seven to eight minutes) and brown, take out the waffle and place on a cooling rack. In a couple of minutes it will further crisp up and will be ready to serve.

8. Similarly make the remaining two waffles.

CUCUMBER AND AVOCADO "ROSES" (SNACK)

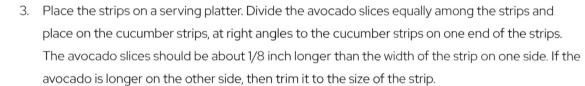

Number of servings:
2

Nutritional values per serving:
Six roses

Calories: 154	**Carbohydrate:** 10g	**Protein:** 3g
Fat: 12g	**Fiber:** 6g	

Ingredients:

- 2 medium English cucumbers, trimmed (do not peel)
- Salt to taste
- 1 avocado, peeled, pitted, cut into thin slices
- 2 teaspoons sesame seeds

Directions:

1. Take a vegetable peeler and peel each cucumber into six long strips. Make three strips from two opposite sides (from each side) so that you will not peel the seeds along.
2. Place the strips on paper towels. Dab with another paper towel on the top of the strips.
3. Place the strips on a serving platter. Divide the avocado slices equally among the strips and place on the cucumber strips, at right angles to the cucumber strips on one end of the strips. The avocado slices should be about 1/8 inch longer than the width of the strip on one side. If the avocado is longer on the other side, then trim it to the size of the strip.
4. Now roll up the strips. Place them upright on a serving platter. These are your roses with avocado in between as the petals.
5. Dust salt over the roses on top. Sprinkle sesame seeds on the roses and serve.

JACKFRUIT PHILLY CHEESESTEAK SANDWICH (LUNCH)

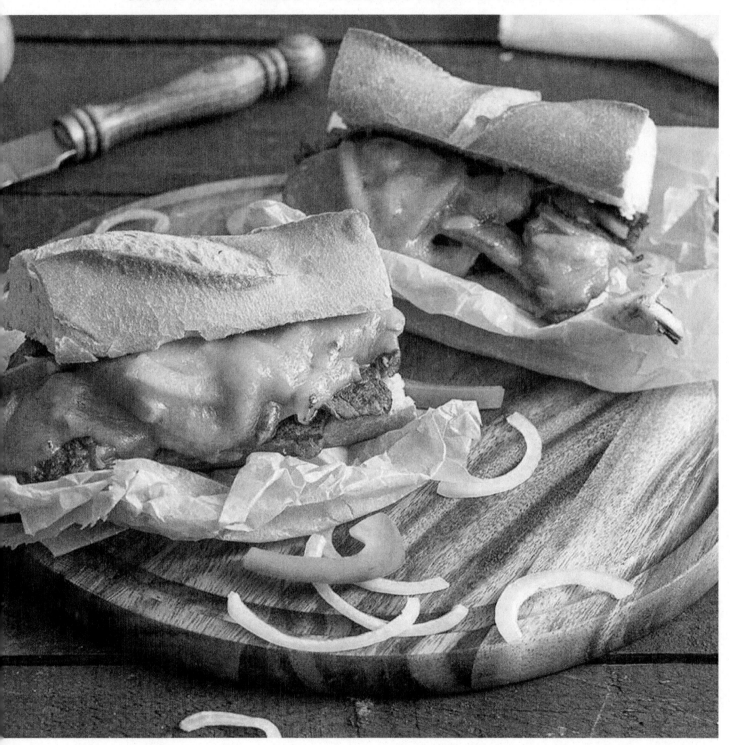

Number of servings:

2

Nutritional values per serving:

Calories: 448	Carbohydrate: 62g	Protein: 8g
Fat: 21g	Fiber: 11g	

Ingredients:

- 1 tablespoon extra-virgin olive oil, divided
- 1 can (20 ounces) jackfruit in brine, drained, rinsed well
- ¼ teaspoon onion powder
- ¼ teaspoon celery seeds
- Pepper to taste
- ½ tablespoon chickpea flour
- Salt to taste
- Cayenne pepper to taste
- ¼ teaspoon paprika
- 2 tablespoons vegetable broth
- ½ tablespoon balsamic vinegar
- 2 tablespoons vegan mayonnaise
- 1 small onion, sliced
- ¼ teaspoon garlic powder +
- extra for the rolls
- 1 tablespoon gluten-free vegan Worcestershire sauce
- 2 whole wheat dinner rolls, split
- ½ cup shredded vegan cheddar cheese

Directions:

1. Set the temperature of the oven to 350°F and preheat the oven. Prepare a baking sheet by lining it with parchment paper.
2. Place a skillet over medium heat. Add ½ tablespoon oil. Once the oil is hot, add onion and sauté until translucent.
3. Lower the heat and cook until golden brown. Stir occasionally. Remove onto a plate.
4. Make sure that you rinse the jackfruit really well; else the dish will be very salty.
5. Dry the jackfruit by placing it over a kitchen towel. Cut the jackfruit into small pieces and add into a bowl.
6. Add spices, celery seeds, and salt and mix until well coated.
7. Place a skillet over medium-high heat. Add jackfruit and dry-roast it for about five minutes. Stir occasionally.
8. Add ½ tablespoon oil into the skillet and mix well. Stir in the browned onions.
9. Add chickpea flour and mix until well coated.
10. Pour broth, vinegar and Worcestershire sauce into the skillet and mix well.
11. Reduce the heat to medium heat and cook until the jackfruit is tender. Stir occasionally.
12. Turn off the heat. When cool enough to handle, shred the jackfruit with a pair of forks and place on the baking sheet, in a single layer.
13. Place the baking sheet in the oven for 15 minutes. This step of baking is to make the jackfruit chewy like meat.
14. Spread one tablespoon mayonnaise on the bottom part of the dinner rolls and place on the baking sheet. Dust with garlic powder. Divide the jackfruit equally and place on the bottom half of the rolls. Sprinkle cheese on top.
15. Turn the oven on to broil mode. Place the baking sheet in the oven. Broil for a couple of minutes.
16. Cover with the top half of the rolls and serve immediately.

RATATOUILLE WITH WHITE BEANS AND POLENTA (DINNER)

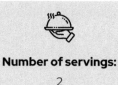

	Nutritional values per serving:		
Number of servings: 2	**Calories:** 458 **Fat:** 25g	**Carbohydrate:** 50g **Fiber:** 10g	**Protein:** 12g

Ingredients:

- 2 ½ tablespoons extra-virgin olive oil, divided
- ½ medium red bell pepper, deseeded, chopped
- ½ small eggplant, cut into ½ inch pieces
- 1 medium zucchini, halved lengthwise and cut into ½ moons
- 1 cup halved cherry or grape tomatoes
- ½ teaspoon Italian seasoning
- ¼ teaspoon ground pepper or to taste
- 1/8 cup pine nuts, roasted
- ½ large onion, chopped
- 2 cloves garlic, minced
- Kosher salt to taste
- ½ can (from a 15 ounces can) unsalted white beans, rinsed
- 1/8 cup slivered sun dried tomatoes
- ½ tablespoons capers, rinsed, chopped
- ½ tube (from a 16-18 ounces tube) prepared polenta, cut into four rounds

Directions:

1. Pour ½ tablespoon oil into a pot and let it heat over medium heat. When the oil is hot, add onion, salt and bell pepper. Cook until the vegetables are a bit tender
2. Stir in the garlic and sauté for a few seconds until you get a nice aroma. Remove the vegetables with a slotted spoon and place in a large bowl.
3. Pour ½ tablespoon oil into the pot. Once the oil is hot, add eggplant and a bit of salt and cook until brown spots appear at a few places on the eggplant pieces. Transfer the eggplant pieces into the bowl of onions.
4. Add ½ tablespoon oil into the pot. Add zucchini and a little salt once the oil is hot and cook until a few brown spots appear on the zucchini pieces.
5. Add tomatoes, beans, sun dried tomatoes, pepper, and Italian seasoning and mix well.
6. Lower the heat and cook until the vegetables are soft. Remove from heat and add capers. Also add the eggplant and onion and mix well.
7. Meanwhile, place a nonstick skillet over medium heat. Add remaining oil. When the oil is hot, place polenta rounds. Cook until the underside is golden brown. Flip sides and cook the other side until golden brown. Remove onto a plate.
8. Divide the ratatouille among two plates. Place two polenta rounds in each. Garnish with pine nuts and serve.

CHUNKY MEDITERRANEAN TOMATO SOUP (SIDE DISH)

Nutritional values per serving:

Number of servings:	Calories:	212	Carbohydrate:	24g	Protein:	11g
2	Fat:	7g	Fiber:	6g		

Ingredients:

- ½ package (from a 14.5 ounces package) frozen grilled mixed vegetables
- 5-6 fresh basil leaves, chopped
- ½ vegetable bouillon cube

- 1 tablespoon chopped garlic
- 1 can (from a 14.5 ounces can) chopped tomatoes
- 2 cups water

To serve:
- 2 slices rye bread
- 3.5 ounces ricotta
- 1 teaspoon minced basil
- 1 teaspoon minced chives

Directions:

1. Place a soup pot over medium-high heat. Add garlic and half the mixed vegetables and until slightly soft.
2. Add tomatoes, basil, vegetable bouillon, and water and mix well. Cook for about five minutes.
3. Blend the mixture with an immersion blender until very smooth.
4. Stir in remaining frozen vegetables and cook until the vegetables are tender.
5. Turn off the heat and serve in soup bowls.
6. Combine ricotta, basil, and chives in a bowl. Spread this mixture over the bread slices.

TUESDAY

GLUTEN-FREE QUICHE LORRAINE (BREAKFAST)

Nutritional values per serving:
½ the quiche

Number of servings:	Calories:	574	Carbohydrate:	14g	Protein:	18g
2	Fat:	52g	Fiber:	4g		

Ingredients:

For filling:
- 1 slice bacon
- 1 ounce Gruyere cheese, shredded
- Yolk of a small egg
- 1 small egg

- Pepper to taste
- ½ medium onion, diced
- 6 tablespoons heavy cream
- Salt to taste
- ½ scallion, chopped

For crust:
- ¾ cup almond flour
- ¾ tablespoon unsalted butter, melted
- Salt to taste
- White of a small egg

Directions:

1. Cook bacon in a pan until crisp. Remove bacon with a slotted spoon and place on a plate lined with paper towels.
2. Set the temperature of the oven to 350°F and preheat the oven.
3. Add onion into the same skillet and cook until soft. Turn off the heat and let the onion cool.
4. Add cream, yolk, egg, nutmeg, pepper, and salt into a bowl and whisk well.
5. To make crust: Combine almond flour and salt in a bowl. Add butter and cut it into the flour with a fork or pastry cutter.
6. Add egg white and mix until the mixture comes together when you press it.
7. Take a small pie pan of about 5-6 inches and place the crust mixture in the pan. Press it well onto the bottom as well as sides of the pan.
8. Scatter bacon on the crust. Sprinkle cheese over the bacon. Spoon the egg mixture over the cheese.
9. Scatter scallion on top. Place the pie pan in the oven and bake until the top is set and the crust turns brown, about 30 minutes.
10. Take out the quiche and cool for 15 minutes. Cut into two halves and serve.

RASPBERRY SMOOTHIE (SNACK)

Nutritional values per serving:
One glass

Number of servings:	Calories:	155	Carbohydrate:	30g	Protein:	7g
2	Fat:	2g	Fiber:	9g		

Ingredients:

- 2 cups frozen raspberries
- 1 cup unsweetened vanilla almond milk
- 12 ounces vanilla Greek yogurt

Directions:

1. Add berries, milk, yogurt, honey and oats into a blender.
2. Blend until you get a smooth texture.
3. Pour into two glasses and serve.

GREEK SALAD WITH EDAMAME (LUNCH)

Nutritional values per serving:
2 ¾ cups

Number of servings:	Calories:	344	Carbohydrate:	19,9g	Protein:	17,7g
2	Fat:	23,3g	Fiber:	8,8g		

Ingredients:

For dressing:
- 2 tablespoons red wine vinegar
- Salt to taste
- 1 ½ tablespoons extra-virgin olive oil
- Pepper to taste

For salad:
- 8 ounces frozen shelled edamame, thawed
- ¼ cucumber, peeled, sliced
- 1/8 cup thinly sliced fresh basil
- 1/8 cup thinly sliced onion
- 4 cups chopped romaine lettuce
- ½ cup halved cherry tomatoes
- ¼ cup crumbled feta cheese
- 1/8 cup sliced kalamata olives

Directions:

1. Whisk together all the dressing ingredients in a bowl. Add all the salad ingredients and toss well.
2. Serve.

JALAPEÑO POPPER BURGERS (DINNER)

	Nutritional values per serving:					
Number of servings: 2	**Calories:**	458	**Carbohydrate:**	28,6g	**Protein:**	32,8g
	Fat:	23,5g	**Fiber:**	3,4g		

Ingredients:

- 1.5 ounces reduced-fat cream cheese, softened
- ½ medium jalapeño pepper, deseeded, chopped

- Kosher salt to taste
- 2 tablespoons ketchup
- 6 tablespoons shredded spicy cheese like pepper

- Jack
- ½ pound ground sirloin
- 2 whole-wheat hamburger buns

Directions:

1. You can grill the burgers on a preheated grill or a preheated grill pan.
2. To make cheese discs: Add spicy cheese, cream cheese, and jalapeño in a bowl and mash with a fork. Mix it up well.
3. Make two equal portions of the mixture and shape into discs.
4. Make two equal portions of the meat and shape into burgers of about ½ inch thick. Sprinkle salt over the burgers.
5. Cook the burgers on the chosen method for about 3-4 minutes on each side. Now lay a cheese disc on each burger and cook for a couple of minutes until the cheese melts or until the internal temperature in the center of the burger shows 160°F.
6. Toast the buns on the grill to the desired doneness.
7. Place burgers over the bottom half of the buns. Spread a tablespoon of ketchup on each. Cover with the top half of the buns and serve.

WEDNESDAY

CAULIFLOWER OMELET (BREAKFAST)

Nutritional values per serving:
One omelet

| **Number of servings:** | **Calories:** | 373 | **Carbohydrate:** 11,2g | **Protein:** | 16,6g |
| 2 | **Fat:** | 30,3g | **Fiber:** 5g | | |

Ingredients:

- 1 head cauliflower florets, cut into small florets
- 4 large eggs
- 1 teaspoon water
- Freshly ground pepper to taste
- Paprika to taste
- 4 teaspoons oil
- Kosher salt to taste
- 12-15 fresh basil leaves, torn

Directions:

1. Set the temperature of the oven to 400°F and preheat the oven.
2. Place the cauliflower florets on a baking sheet. Spray some cooking spray over the cauliflower florets.
3. Place the baking sheet in the oven and set the timer for 25-30 minutes or until the cauliflower florets are brown and tender.
4. Place a medium size skillet over medium heat. Pour two teaspoons of oil into the skillet and swirl the pan to spread oil. Let the oil heat.
5. Meanwhile, whisk eggs in a bowl with pepper, salt, and water.
6. Pour half the eggs into the skillet. Let the eggs cook for about a minute. Scatter half the cauliflower florets over the eggs.
7. When the omelet is nearly cooked and the underside is golden brown, turn the omelet over and cook the other side as well.
8. Remove the omelet onto a plate and serve garnished with paprika.
9. Cook the other omelet similarly.

SPICY MUSHROOM WRAP (SNACK)

	Nutritional values per serving: One wrap		
Number of servings: 3	**Calories:** 251 **Fat:** 10g	**Carbohydrate:** 31g **Fiber:** 3,9g	**Protein:** 11g

Ingredients:

For filling:

- 1 tablespoon olive oil
- 1 clove garlic, minced
- Salt to taste
- 7 ounces baby button mushrooms, sliced

- ½ medium red onion, sliced
- Pepper to taste

For dip:

- 2.5 ounces Greek yogurt
- ¼ teaspoon chili flakes
- ¼ teaspoon minced garlic

- ¼ teaspoon dried thyme

To assemble:

- 3 whole-wheat tortillas
- 1 medium tomato, sliced
- ½ cup baby spinach
- ½ chili, sliced

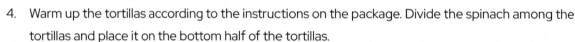

Directions:

1. Pour a tablespoon of oil into a skillet. Heat it over medium heat.
2. When oil is hot, add onion and garlic and cook for about a minute. Stir in mushrooms and cook until brown. Add salt and pepper to taste and turn off the heat.
3. To make dip: Combine all the ingredients for dip in a bowl. Cover and set it aside in the refrigerator until you need to serve.
4. Warm up the tortillas according to the instructions on the package. Divide the spinach among the tortillas and place it on the bottom half of the tortillas.
5. Place equal tomato slices and chilies over the spinach. Spread mushrooms over the tomato slices.
6. Roll the tortillas and place it on a serving platter with the seam side facing down. Cut each into two halves and serve.

SPINACH AND ARTICHOKE SALAD WITH PARMESAN VINAIGRETTE (LUNCH)

Number of servings:
2

Nutritional values per serving:

Calories:	324	**Carbohydrate:** 11,9g	**Protein:** 16g
Fat:	23,8g	**Fiber:** 3,8g	

Ingredients:

- ½ can (from a 15 ounces can) quartered artichoke hearts, drained, rinsed well
- 3 cups packed baby spinach
- 1/8 cup chopped unsalted pistachios

- 3 hard boiled eggs, peeled, quartered

For Parmesan vinaigrette:
- 1 tablespoon lemon juice
- 1 tablespoon grated Parmesan cheese
- ½ teaspoon Dijon mustard

- Pepper to taste
- 2 tablespoons extra-virgin olive oil
- 1 tablespoon minced shallot
- 1 teaspoon finely chopped fresh chives
- Salt to taste

Directions:

1. To make Parmesan vinaigrette: Whisk together all the vinaigrette ingredients in a bowl. Cover the bowl and chill until use.
2. Place artichoke hearts over a kitchen towel for about 15 minutes to drain off any water.
3. Divide equally artichoke hearts, spinach, eggs, and pistachios into two bowls. Toss well.
4. Divide the dressing among the bowls. Toss well and serve.

STEAMED CARROTS WITH GARLIC-GINGER BUTTER (SIDE DISH)

	Nutritional values per serving:				
Number of servings:	**Calories:**	69	**Carbohydrate:**	10,3g	**Protein:**	0,9g
2	**Fat:**	3g	**Fiber:**	3,4g		

Ingredients:

- 1 clove garlic, minced
- ½ tablespoon butter
- ½ tablespoon chopped cilantro
- ½ tablespoon fresh lime juice
- ½ pound baby carrots with tops, peeled
- ½ teaspoon minced, peeled, fresh ginger
- ¼ teaspoon grated lime zest
- Salt to taste

Directions:

1. Set up your steaming equipment and place the carrots in the steaming basket.
2. Steam for 10-12 minutes.
3. Melt butter in a nonstick pan over medium heat. When butter melts, add ginger and garlic and stir-fry for a few seconds until you get a nice aroma.
4. Add carrots and mix well. Add salt to taste. Garnish with cilantro and serve.

CHICKEN WITH RICE AND BLACK-EYED PEAS (DINNER) VINAIGRETTE (LUNCH)

Nutritional values per serving:

Number of servings:	Calories:	571	Carbohydrate:	48g	Protein:	49g
2	Fat:	18g	Fiber:	10g		

Ingredients:

- ½ tablespoon olive oil
- 2 chicken thighs (1.1 pounds), skinless
- ½ tablespoon curry powder or to taste
- 2 large tomatoes, chopped
- 1 clove garlic, chopped
- 1 red onion, sliced
- ½ tablespoon fresh thyme leaves

- ½ teaspoon ground allspice
- ½ red chili, deseed if desired, sliced
- 1 teaspoon vegetable bouillon
- Salt to taste
- 1 cup water

For rice and black-eyed peas:
- 2.2 ounces brown basmati rice

- 10.1 ounces water
- 1 clove garlic, chopped
- ½ teaspoon vegetable bouillon
- ½ red onion, chopped
- ½ tablespoon chopped fresh thyme leaves + extra to garnish
- ½ can (from a 14.5 ounces can) black-eyed peas

Directions:

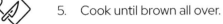

1. To cook rice and black-eyed peas: Combine rice, onion, vegetable bouillon, thyme, garlic, and water in a saucepan.
2. Place the saucepan over medium heat. When water starts boiling, lower the heat and cook covered until dry and rice is cooked.
3. Meanwhile cook the chicken: Pour oil into a nonstick pan and heat it over medium heat.
4. Combine curry powder, thyme, allspice, and thyme in a bowl. Sprinkle this mixture all over the chicken and place it in the pan.
5. Cook until brown all over.
6. Add tomatoes, red chili, bouillon, and garlic and mix well. Add water and mix well.
7. Keep the pan covered and cook until the chicken is well-cooked.
8. When rice is cooked, add beans and mix well. Turn off the heat and let it remain covered for 10 minutes.
9. Divide the rice among two serving plates. Divide chicken and gravy equally and spoon over the rice.
10. Serve hot along with steamed carrots with garlic ginger butter.

THURSDAY

SUMMER SKILLET VEGETABLE AND EGG SCRAMBLE (BREAKFAST)

Number of servings:
2

Nutritional values per serving:
1 ½ cups

Calories:	254	Carbohydrate:	19,2g	Protein:	12,4g
Fat:	14,2g	Fiber:	4,3g		

Ingredients:

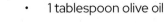

- 1 tablespoon olive oil
- 2 cups mixed sliced vegetables (zucchini, bell peppers, and mushrooms)
- ½ teaspoon minced fresh
- herbs of your choice
- 1 cup packed baby spinach or kale
- 6 ounces baby potatoes, thinly sliced
- 2 small scallions, thinly sliced (keep the green and white parts separate)
- 3 large eggs or two large eggs + two

Directions:

1. Place a nonstick skillet over medium heat. Add oil. When oil is hot, add potatoes and cook covered, until slightly tender.
2. Stir in vegetables and the whites of the scallions and mix well. Do not cover the pan now.
3. Once the potatoes are cooked, add fresh herbs and mix well.
4. Push the vegetables to one side of the pan. Place scallion greens in the middle of the pan. Pour egg and stir often until the eggs are soft cooked.
5. Add greens and mix it all up, eggs, greens, and vegetables.
6. Add salt to taste. Mix well and turn off the heat.
7. Serve hot.

BLUEBERRY PASSION FRUIT SMOOTHIE (SNACK)

Nutritional values per serving:

Number of servings:	Calories:	124	Carbohydrate:	29,9g	Protein:	3,5g
2	Fat:	0,7g	Fiber:	3,5g		

Ingredients:

- ½ cup plain fat-free yogurt
- Ice cubes, as required
- 1 teaspoon honey
- ½ ripe banana, sliced
- ¼ cup passion fruit nectar
- ¾ teaspoon toasted wheat
- germ
- 6 ounces frozen blueberries

Directions:

1. Place yogurt, ice, honey, banana, passion fruit nectar, wheat germ, and blueberries in a blender.
2. Blend until you get a smooth mixture.
3. Pour into two glasses and serve.

CHOPPED COBB SALAD (LUNCH)

Nutritional values per serving:

Number of servings:	Calories:	481	Carbohydrate:	67,6g	Protein:	17,3g
2	Fat:	16,7g	Fiber:	13,4g		

Ingredients:

- 6 cups chopped iceberg lettuce
- 2 stalks celery, diced
- 2 hard boiled eggs, peeled,
- diced
- 4 tablespoons honey mustard vinaigrette
- 2 roasted chicken thighs,
- diced
- 2 carrots, diced
- 1/8 cup crumbled blue cheese

Directions:

1. Place chicken, eggs, blue cheese, and vegetables in a salad bowl and toss well.
2. Pour dressing over the salad. Toss well. Divide equally into two plates and serve.

CHICKEN PARMESAN AND VEGGIE SKILLET (DINNER) VINAIGRETTE (LUNCH)

Number of servings:	Nutritional values per serving:				
2	Calories:	747	Carbohydrate: 62g	Protein:	67g
	Fat:	25g	Fiber: 10g		

Ingredients:

- 4 tablespoons all-purpose flour
- Black pepper to taste
- ¼ cup plain breadcrumbs
- 2 boneless, skinless chicken breasts
- ½ teaspoon red pepper

- flakes
- 2 cups canned crushed tomatoes with its juice
- 2 tablespoons chopped basil
- Salt to taste
- 2 large eggs, beaten

- 4 teaspoons olive oil
- 1 teaspoon minced garlic
- 2.4 pounds eggplant, diced
- 2 slices fresh mozzarella cheese

Directions:

1. You need to set the temperature of the oven to 375°F and preheat the oven.
2. Mix together flour, salt and pepper in a shallow bowl.
3. Add breadcrumbs into another bowl.
4. First dredge the chicken in flour. Next dip the chicken in egg. Shaking off excess egg, dredge the chicken in breadcrumbs and place on a plate.
5. Place an ovenproof skillet over medium heat. Add three teaspoons of oil. When oil is hot, place chicken in the pan and cook for three minutes or until the underside is golden brown.
6. Turn the chicken over and cook the other side until golden brown.
7. Take out the chicken from the pan and place on a plate.
8. Pour remaining oil into the pan. Add eggplants, garlic, and red pepper flakes and mix well. Cook until tender.
9. Add salt, crushed tomatoes, and pepper and mix well. Turn off the heat.
10. Place chicken over the eggplant. Lay the mozzarella slices over the chicken.
11. Shift the skillet into the oven and bake for a few minutes until the chicken melts.

FRIDAY

AVOCADO AND KALE OMELET (BREAKFAST)

Nutritional values per serving:

Number of servings:	Calories:	339	Carbohydrate:	8,6g	Protein:	15g
2	Fat:	28,1g	Fiber:	4,4g		

Ingredients:

- 4 large eggs
- Salt to taste
- 2 cups chopped kale
- 1/8 cup chopped fresh cilantro
- Crushed red pepper to taste
- ½ avocado, peeled, pitted, sliced
- 2 teaspoons low-fat milk
- 4 teaspoons extra-virgin olive oil, divided
- 2 tablespoons lime juice
- 2 teaspoons unsalted sunflower seeds
- Salt to taste

Directions:

1. Crack eggs into a bowl. Add salt and milk and whisk well.
2. Pour one teaspoon of oil into a small, nonstick skillet and place the skillet over medium heat.
3. Pour half the egg mixture into the pan and cook until the edges are set and the center is not well cooked. Carefully turn the omelet over and cook for about ½ a minute.
4. Slide the omelet onto a plate.
5. Make the other omelet similarly (steps 2-4).
6. Place kale, cilantro, and sunflower seeds in a bowl. Drizzle two teaspoons of oil and lemon juice over the kale. Add salt and crushed red pepper and toss well.
7. Divide the kale equally and spread it over the omelets. Divide the avocado slices among the omelets and serve.

SWEET POTATO TOTS WITH JALAPEÑO GARLIC RANCH DIPPING SAUCE (SNACK)

	Nutritional values per serving: 12-15 tots		
Number of servings: 2	**Calories:** 235 **Fat:** 6,8g	**Carbohydrate:** 35g **Fiber:** 4g	**Protein:** 10g

Ingredients:

For sweet potato tots:

- 3 small sweet potatoes, pricked all over with a fork
- Kosher salt to taste
- 6 tablespoons panko breadcrumbs
- ½ teaspoon ground cinnamon, divided
- 2 tablespoons almond meal
- 1 egg white, beaten

For jalapeño garlic ranch dipping sauce:

- ¼ cup 2% Greek yogurt
- 1 tablespoon low-fat mayonnaise
- ½ clove garlic, sliced
- 1 tablespoon chopped parsley
- 1 tablespoon chopped chives

- Freshly ground pepper to taste
- 1 ½ tablespoons low-fat buttermilk
- ½ tablespoon Dijon mustard
- ½ jalapeño, deseeded, sliced
- Salt to taste

Directions:

1. Set the temperature of the oven to 400°F and preheat the oven. Line a baking sheet with foil.
2. Place the sweet potatoes on the baking sheet. Set the timing for about 40 minutes or until soft.
3. Take out the baking sheet from the oven and let the sweet potatoes cool.
4. Peel the sweet potatoes and mash it adding salt and ¼ teaspoon cinnamon.
5. Chill for about 20 minutes.
6. Mix together almond meal, ¼ teaspoon cinnamon, panko breadcrumbs, and salt.
7. Make small tots of the sweet potato mixture.
8. Spray the baking sheet with some oil.
9. Dip the tots in egg white, one at a time. Shaking off excess egg, dredge the tots in the panko mixture and place on the baking sheet.
10. Spray some cooking spray on top of the tots and place the baking sheet in the oven for about 45 minutes. Turn the tots every 15 minutes for even browning.
11. To make dressing: Place all the dressing ingredients in a blender and blend until smooth.
12. Pour into a bowl and serve with sweet potato tots.

LINGUINE WITH CREAMY WHITE CLAM SAUCE (LUNCH)

Nutritional values per serving:
1 ¼ cups

Number of servings:	Calories:	421	Carbohydrate:	51,9g	Protein:	21,5g
2	Fat:	16,6g	Fiber:	7,8g		

Ingredients:

- 4 ounces whole-wheat linguine
- 1 ½ tablespoons extra-virgin olive oil
- 1/8 teaspoon crushed red pepper
- Salt to taste
- 1/8 cup chopped basil + extra to garnish
- ½ container (from a 16 ounces container) chopped clams or one can (10 ounces) whole baby clams
- 2 cloves garlic, chopped
- ½ tablespoon lemon juice
- ½ large tomato, chopped
- 1 tablespoon heavy cream or half and half

Directions:

1. Cook pasta following the directions given on the package.
2. Retain about 2/3 cup of the liquid from the clam.
3. Pour oil into a skillet and heat over medium-high heat. When oil is hot, add garlic and cook for a few seconds until you get a nice aroma.
4. Stir in crushed red pepper. Pour the retained clam liquid, salt, and lemon juice and cook for a couple of minutes.
5. Stir in tomatoes and clams. Let it come to a boil. Turn off the heat after a minute.
6. Add basil and cream and mix well. Stir in pasta.
7. Sprinkle basil on top and serve.

TANGY TROUT WITH GARDEN SALAD (DINNER)

	Nutritional values per serving:					
Number of servings: 2	**Calories:**	583	**Carbohydrate:**	6g	**Protein:**	50g
	Fat:	40g	**Fiber:**	2g		

Ingredients:

- 1 lemon, cut into thin slices
- Juice of a lemon
- 2 rainbow trout's, gutted, rinsed (12 ounces each)
- ¼ cup Greek yogurt

- 8 green beans, stringed, cut into thin slices on the diagonal
- Few sprigs dill
- ¼ cup chopped dill

- 4 tablespoons olive oil + extra to grease
- 1 clove garlic, minced
- 6 radishes, cut into thin round slices

Directions:

1. Set the temperature of the oven to 390°F and preheat the oven. Line a baking sheet with foil or grease the baking sheet.
2. Divide the lemon slices equally and stuff it into the cavity of the trout's. Also stuff the dill sprigs and place them on the baking sheet.
3. Score the trout at 3-4 places. Pour ½ tablespoon oil on top of each trout.
4. Sprinkle salt and pepper to taste and place it in the oven for 15 minutes or until cooked through.
5. To make yogurt sauce: Combine dill and yogurt in a bowl. Add a teaspoon of lemon juice, salt, and pepper and stir. Cover and set aside for a while for the flavors to mingle.
6. Blanch the beans in a pot of boiling water until crisp as well as tender. Drain and place the beans in a bowl.
7. Also add garlic and radish into the bowl of beans and mix well.
8. To serve: Place a trout on each plate. Divide the salad among the plates. Drizzle remaining lemon juice over the trout's. Serve with yogurt dill sauce.

SATURDAY

SAVORY BREAKFAST SALAD (BREAKFAST)

Nutritional values per serving:

Number of servings: 1	**Calories:** 523 **Fat:** 37,9g	**Carbohydrate:** 57,6g **Fiber:** 15g	**Protein:** 7,5g

Ingredients:

For sweet potatoes:
- 4 small sweet potatoes,
- Salt to taste
- ½ tablespoon olive oil or avocado oil
- Pepper to taste

For salad and serving:
- 2 cups mixed greens
- 2 tablespoons hummus
- Chopped parsley to garnish
- ½ medium ripe avocado, peeled, pitted, chopped
- 1 tablespoon hemp seeds

(optional)
For dressing:
- 1 ½ tablespoons lemon juice
- Salt to taste
- ½ tablespoon extra-virgin olive oil
- Pepper to taste

Directions:

1. Pour oil into a skillet and let it heat over medium heat.
2. When the oil is hot, add sweet potatoes and stir. Season with salt and pepper and spread it in a single layer.
3. Cover the pan and cook for about three to four minutes or until the underside is golden brown. Turn the sweet potatoes over and similarly cook until they are golden brown all over and cooked through inside.
4. To make dressing: Whisk together oil, lemon juice, pepper, and salt in a bowl.
5. To assemble: Place mixed greens on a plate. Place sweet potatoes over the greens.
6. Scatter blueberries, avocado, hemp seeds, and parsley over the greens. Place the bowl of dressing alongside and serve.

NUTTY PARMESAN HERB SCONES (SNACK)SAUCE (SNACK)

	Nutritional values per serving:			
Number of servings:	**Calories:**	196	**Carbohydrate:** 14g	**Protein:** 7g
6	**Fat:**	12,7g	**Fiber:** 3g	

Ingredients:

- ½ cup old fashioned rolled oats
- 2 tablespoons extra-virgin olive oil
- 1 large egg
- 1/3 cup chopped, toasted walnuts
- ½ tablespoon chopped
- fresh thyme
- 1/8 teaspoon baking powder
- 1.5 ounces Parmesan cheese
- 1/8 cup warm water
- ½ tablespoon brown sugar
- 2 ¼ ounces white whole-
- wheat flour
- 1 tablespoon ground flaxseed
- ¼ teaspoon kosher salt or to taste
- 1/8 teaspoon black pepper

Directions:

1. Set the temperature of the oven to 350°F and preheat the oven. Prepare a baking sheet by lining it with parchment paper.
2. Mix together oats and water in a mixing bowl.
3. Crack egg into a bowl. Add sugar and oil and whisk well.
4. Pour the egg mixture into the bowl of oats and stir.
5. Add all the dry ingredients into another bowl, i.e. flour, flaxseeds, nuts, thyme, pepper, baking soda, salt, and cheese.
6. Add the mixture of dry ingredients into the bowl of oat mixture and stir using a fork.
7. You will get dough that is sticky to touch.
8. Dust your hands with flour and knead the dough twice or trice and no longer.
9. Make six equal portions of the dough and form each into a triangle of ¼ inch thick.
10. Place them on a baking sheet, making sure to leave sufficient gaps between them.
11. Place the baking dish in the oven and set the timer for about 18 minutes. Bake until golden brown.

GRILLED CHICKEN TACOS WITH SLAW AND LIME CREMA (LUNCH)

	Nutritional values per serving: Two tacos				
Number of servings: 2	**Calories:** **Fat:**	339 12,1g	**Carbohydrate:** **Fiber:**	31,4g 6,3g	**Protein:** 27,7g

Ingredients:

- 1 ½ cups thinly sliced red cabbage
- ¼ cup thinly sliced scallions
- ½ teaspoon salt, divided
- 1/8 cup chopped cilantro
- ¾ tablespoon olive oil
- 4 corn tortillas (8 inches each), warmed
- Lime wedges to serve (optional)
- ½ cup julienned carrots
- 2 tablespoons fresh lime juice, divided
- 3 tablespoons low-fat sour cream
- 4 chicken tenders
- ½ tablespoon chili powder or to taste
- ½ jalapeno pepper, thinly sliced

Directions:

1. To make slaw: Place carrots, cabbage, and scallions in a bowl and toss well. Stir in a tablespoon of lime juice and ¼ teaspoon salt.
2. To make lime crema: Whisk together sour cream, one tablespoon lime juice, and cilantro in another bowl.
3. Place a grill pan over high heat. Spray the pan with some cooking spray. Brush oil over the chicken tenders and place it in the hot pan.
4. Cook on both the sides for 6-8 minutes on each side or until the internal temperature in the center of the thickest part of the meat shows 165°F on the meat thermometer.
5. Distribute equal quantities of chicken over the tortillas. Divide the slaw and lime crema equally and place over the chicken.
6. Sprinkle cilantro and serve along with lime wedges if using.

SEARED SESAME TUNA BOWLS (DINNER)

	Nutritional values per serving: One bowl				
Number of servings: 2	**Calories:** 534	**Carbohydrate:** 42g	**Protein:** 46,7g
	Fat: 19,2g	**Fiber:** 6,5g	

Ingredients:

- 1 tablespoon toasted sesame seeds (black or white)
- 2 ahi tuna fillets, (5 ounces each)
- 1 ½ tablespoons rice vinegar
- ¾ teaspoon grated ginger
- ¼ teaspoon grated fresh garlic
- 2 teaspoons canola oil, divided
- 2 tablespoons tahini
- 1 ½ tablespoons low-sodium soy sauce
- ½ teaspoon toasted sesame oil

For the bowls:

- 1 cup cooked brown rice
- ½ cup cooked, shelled edamame
- ¼ cup thinly sliced scallions
- Lime juice to drizzle (optional)
- 1 cup thinly sliced English cucumber (cut into ½ moon slices)
- ¼ cup chopped cilantro
- 1/8 cup pickled ginger

Directions:

1. Set the temperature of the oven to 375°F and preheat the oven.
2. Using ½ teaspoon of oil, brush it on one side of each fillet.
3. Dredge tuna in sesame seeds, on the oiled side.
4. Pour 1 ½ teaspoons oil into an ovenproof skillet and place it over medium-high heat.
5. When oil is hot, place tuna in the pan, with the sesame seed side facing on top.
6. Cook for about four minutes, until the underside is crispy. Turn off the heat and shift the skillet into the oven, on the top rack.
7. Bake until the top is golden brown and the temperature of the meat in the thickest part of the tuna shows 140°F.
8. Place tahini, soy sauce, sesame oil, vinegar, ginger, and garlic in a bowl and whisk well.
9. Take two bowls and place ½ cup rice in each bowl. Divide equally the cucumber, scallions, edamame, pickled ginger, and cilantro and place it over the rice.
10. Place a fillet on top in each bowl. Drizzle the tahini sauce mixture on top and serve.

S U N D A Y

MEDITERRANEAN EGG CASSEROLE (BREAKFAST)

Nutritional values per serving:

Number of servings: 4	**Calories:** 360 **Fat:** 20g	**Carbohydrate:** 7g **Fiber:** 3g	**Protein:** 24g

Ingredients:

- ½ tablespoon vegetable oil
- ¼ cup chopped red bell pepper
- 1 cup chopped fresh baby spinach
- ¾ cup crumbled feta cheese
- 3 tablespoons pitted, halved kalamata olives
- 5 eggs
- ¼ teaspoon red pepper flakes
- ¼ teaspoon pepper
- 1/8 cup chopped red onion
- ½ tablespoon minced garlic
- 3 cups cubed French baguette
- ¼ cup shredded Parmesan
- cheese
- 1/8 cup sun-dried tomatoes packed in oil, drained, chopped
- ½ jar (from a six ounces jar) marinated artichoke hearts, drained, chopped
- 1 cup milk
- ¼ teaspoon salt

Directions:

1. Set the temperature of the oven to 375°F and preheat the oven.
2. Prepare a baking dish (8x8 inches) by greasing it with cooking spray.
3. Pour oil into a pan and place the pan over medium heat.
4. Once oil is hot, add onion, garlic, and bell pepper and cook until slightly tender.
5. Stir in spinach and cook until spinach just wilts, about 50-60 seconds. Turn off the heat.
6. Scatter half the baguette on the bottom of the baking dish. Sprinkle ½ cup feta cheese followed by 1/8 cup Parmesan cheese. Next layer with onion mixture followed by artichokes and olives.
7. Next layer should be of sun-dried tomatoes followed by the remaining baguette. Scatter ¼ cup feta cheese on top.
8. Crack eggs into a bowl. Add milk, salt, pepper, and red pepper flakes and whisk well.
9. Drizzle the egg mixture over the casserole and press it with a spatula.
10. Top with 1/8 cup Parmesan cheese.
11. Place the baking dish in the oven and bake until golden brown on top.
12. Let the casserole rest for 10-15 minutes.
13. Serve.

CHOPPED MEDITERRANEAN SALAD (SNACK)

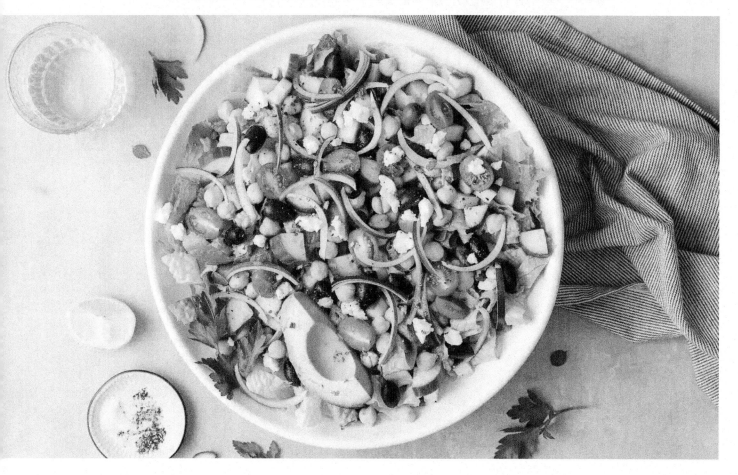

Nutritional values per serving:

Number of servings:	Calories:	288	Carbohydrate:	20g	Protein:	9g
2	Fat:	20g	Fiber:	4g		

Ingredients:

- 1 cucumber, peeled, diced (½ inch dice)
- ½ red onion, thinly sliced
- 2 tomatoes, diced (½ inch dice)
- ¼ cup crumbled feta
- cheese
- 1 tablespoon red wine vinegar
- Freshly ground pepper to taste
- ½ cup pitted, sliced
- kalamata olives
- 1 tablespoon olive oil
- Salt to taste
- ½ tablespoon lemon juice

Directions:

1. Combine cucumber, onion, tomatoes, oil, vinegar, salt, lemon juice, olives, and pepper in a bowl.
2. Serve.

GREEK CHICKEN AND CUCUMBER PITA SANDWICHES WITH YOGURT SAUCE (LUNCH)

	Nutritional values per serving: One half pita sandwich			
Number of servings: 2	**Calories:**	535	**Carbohydrate:** 33,3g	**Protein:** 37,5g
	Fat:	8,6g	**Fiber:** 5,8g	

Ingredients:

- ½ teaspoon grated lemon zest
- 2 ½ teaspoons olive oil, divided
- 1 ½ teaspoons minced garlic
- ½ pound chicken tenders
- Salt to taste
- ½ tablespoon chopped fresh oregano of ½ teaspoon dried oregano
- 1/8 teaspoon crushed red pepper flakes
- ½ English cucumber, halved
- 6 tablespoons nonfat Greek yogurt
- 1 teaspoon chopped fresh dill
- 1 teaspoon chopped fresh dill
- 1 whole-wheat pita bread (6
- ½ inches), halved
- ¼ cup sliced red onion
- 1 tablespoon fresh lemon juice
- ½ teaspoon pepper or to taste
- 2 lettuce leaves
- ½ cup chopped plum tomatoes

Directions:

1. Place lemon juice, lemon zest, oregano, 1 ½ teaspoons oil, crushed red pepper, and one teaspoon garlic in a bowl and whisk well.
2. Stir in the chicken. Cover the bowl and chill for 1-4 hours, to marinate.
3. In the meantime, cut one half of the cucumber into thin slices and grate the other half.
4. To make yogurt sauce: Place grated cucumber in a fine wire mesh strainer. Sprinkle a bit of salt over it and keep the strainer over a bowl for 15 minutes to drain.
5. Now squeeze any extra moisture from the cucumber and add it into a bowl. Add yogurt, pepper, salt, remaining garlic, one teaspoon oil, and herbs and stir. Cover the bowl and chill until use.
6. Set up your grill and preheat it to medium-high heat. Take out the chicken from the marinade and place on the grill and cook for 3-4 minutes on each side or until the internal temperature in the center of the meat in the thickest part shows 165°F on the meat thermometer.
7. To assemble: Apply the sauce inside the pita pockets. Divide equally and fill the chicken, onion, lettuce, cucumber, and tomatoes into the pita pockets.

MEDITERRANEAN FISH CAKES (DINNER)

	Nutritional values per serving:		
	Two fish cakes		
Number of servings:	**Calories:** 560	**Carbohydrate:** 34g	**Protein:** 53,6g
6	**Fat:** 23,2g	**Fiber:** 3,6g	

Ingredients:

- 8 tablespoons olive oil, divided
- 1 medium onion, quartered
- 10 sun-dried tomatoes, chopped
- 2 bunches fresh parsley, chopped
- 2 tablespoons Italian seasoning
- 2 cans (9 ounces each) tuna, drained
- ½ cup all-purpose flour
- 12 ounces fresh bay scallops
- 8 cloves garlic, peeled
- 2 eggs
- 12 basil leaves
- 1 cup breadcrumbs
- 4 fresh hot chili peppers, sliced
- 2 cans (6.5 ounces each) shrimp, drained

Directions:

1. Pour two tablespoons of oil into a large skillet and let it heat over medium-high heat. When oil is hot, add scallops and cook until they are white in color all over. Remove scallops from the pan and place on a plate. Let it cool for a while.
2. Blend together garlic, onion, eggs, sun dried tomatoes, herbs, chilies, and Italian seasoning in the food processor bowl and give short pulses until chopped.
3. Add scallops, tuna, and shrimp and give short pulses until finely chopped.
4. Add breadcrumbs and give short pulses until just combined and a bit sticky but not smooth in texture.
5. Make 12 equal portions of the mixture and shape into patties of about one inch thickness.
6. Keep the patties on a plate and chill for an hour.
7. Pour two tablespoons of oil into a nonstick skillet and let it heat over medium heat. When oil is hot, place 5-6 patties in the pan and cook until the underside is golden brown.
8. Turn the patties over and cook the other side until golden brown.

WEEK 4 – MONDAY

CHOCOLATE CREAM PANCAKE (BREAKFAST)

Nutritional values per serving:
One pancake with ¾ tablespoon chocolate cream

Number of servings:	Calories:	351	Carbohydrate:	40g	Protein:	37g
2	Fat:	5g	Fiber:	5g		

Ingredients:

For the pancakes:

- 1 tablespoon buckwheat flour
- ½ tablespoon ground flax seeds
- ¼ teaspoon baking powder
- 1 tablespoon pea protein
- powder
- ½–1 tablespoon apple cider vinegar
- Stevia to taste
- ½ cup cannellini beans
- ¼ teaspoon olive or canola oil and more if required
- 2 tablespoons water or more if required

For the chocolate cream:

- ½ tablespoon flaxseed oil
- ½ tablespoon cocoa powder
- ½ tablespoon agave nectar

Directions:

1. Add buckwheat flour, pea protein, flax seeds, vinegar, baking powder, stevia and of water into a blender and blend until smooth. If the batter is very thick, add more water, a tablespoon at a time and blend well each time until the consistency you desire is achieved.
2. Place a nonstick pan over medium heat. Add oil. When the oil is hot, add ½ the batter on the pan.
3. When the underside is golden brown, turn the pancake over and cook the other side. Remove the pancake onto a plate.
4. Make the other pancake similarly.
5. To make the chocolate cream: Mix together all the ingredients for chocolate cream in a bowl.
6. Serve warm pancakes with the chocolate cream.

LEMON STRAWBERRY MUFFINS (SNACK)

Number of servings:
3

Nutritional values per serving:
One muffin

Calories:	295	Carbohydrate: 40g	Protein: 8g
Fat:	15g	Fiber: 4g	

Ingredients:

- 1 tablespoon ground chia seeds or chia seeds, divided
- ¼ cup coconut sugar
- ½ tablespoon lemon juice
- 2 ½ tablespoons dairy-free butter

- ¼ cup + one tablespoon non-dairy milk of your choice
- 1 ½ tablespoons water
- ¼ teaspoon baking soda
- ¾ teaspoon baking powder
- A pinch salt

- ¼ cup chopped strawberries
- ¾ cup whole wheat flour
- ¼ cup shelled raw hemp seeds

Directions:

1. Set the temperature of the oven to 375°F and preheat the oven.
2. Grease three muffin cups with some cooking spray.
3. Combine ½ tablespoon chia seeds with water and stir. Let it sit for 15 minutes. This is your flax egg.
4. Add vegan butter and coconut sugar into a mixing bowl. Beat with an electric hand mixer until creamy.
5. Beat in the flax egg. Beat in the lemon juice and milk.
6. Add all the dry ingredients into a bowl, i.e. whole-wheat flour, baking soda, baking powder, hemp seeds, salt, and ½ tablespoon chia seeds and stir. Add into the mixing bowl.
7. Beat until just incorporated, making sure not to overbeat. The batter will be sticky.
8. Add strawberries and fold gently.
9. Divide equally the batter and spoon the batter into the prepared muffin cups.
10. Bake the muffins for about 15-18 minutes or until cooked through. To check if it is cooked, insert a toothpick in the center of a muffin and pull it out. If you find some particles stuck on it, you need to bake for another 5-8 minutes, otherwise turn off the oven and remove the muffin cups.
11. Cool for a few minutes. Run a knife around the edges of the muffins. Invert onto a plate and serve.

CAULIFLOWER CHICKPEA WRAPS (LUNCH)

Nutritional values per serving:
Two wraps

Number of servings:	Calories:	640	Carbohydrate:	98g	Protein:	21g
1	Fat:	23g	Fiber:	11,1g		

Ingredients:

- ¼ inch fresh ginger, minced
- ½ can (14.5 ounces) chickpeas, drained, rinsed
- 4 ounces cauliflower, cut into florets
- 1 tablespoon arrowroot starch
- 2 wraps
- 2 ounces baby spinach

- Salt to taste
- 1 clove garlic, minced
- ½ red onion, thinly sliced
- 1 teaspoon shawarma spice blend
- Juice of ½ lemon
- 1 ½ tablespoons shredded coconut, toasted
- ½ tablespoon olive oil

For cilantro sauce:
- 1/8 cup vegan yogurt
- 1 teaspoon chopped fresh cilantro
- ½ tablespoon lemon juice
- Salt to taste
- Pepper to taste

Directions:

1. Set the temperature of the oven to 375°F and preheat the oven.
2. Prepare a baking sheet by greasing it with a little oil.
3. Add chickpeas, ginger, garlic, lemon juice, onion, shawarma spice blend, salt, arrowroot, cauliflower, and oil into a bowl and toss well.
4. Spread the mixture onto the prepared baking sheet.
5. Place the baking sheet in the oven and bake until the cauliflower is cooked and brown at a few spots.
6. To make cilantro sauce: Add all the ingredients for cilantro sauce into a bowl and whisk well.
7. Cover the bowl and chill until use. It can last for three days.
8. To serve: Warm the tortillas following the instructions on the package.
9. Divide equally the roasted vegetable mixture and spinach and place over the tortillas. Drizzle cilantro sauce over the vegetables. Scatter toasted coconut on top
10. Wrap like a burrito and serve.

CORN AND BEAN CASSEROLE (DINNER)

	Nutritional values per serving:			
Number of servings: 2	**Calories:** 297 **Fat:** 4,9g	**Carbohydrate:** 55,5g **Fiber:** 13,4g	**Protein:** 12,6g	

Ingredients:

- ½ can (from a 15 ounces can) pinto beans, drained, rinsed
- ¼ cup water
- 1 small onion, chopped
- ½ tablespoon ground cumin
- ¾ cup cooked corn kernels
- ¾ cup homemade salsa
- 1 teaspoon canola oil
- ½ tomato, chopped
- 2 medium corn tortillas
- 1 tablespoon Tofutti better than sour cream (vegan sour cream)
- Cooking spray
- Guacamole to serve

Directions:

1. Set the temperature of the oven to 375°F and preheat the oven.
2. Grease a small baking dish (about six inches) with cooking spray.
3. Pour oil into a skillet and heat it over medium heat. Add onion and cook until slightly pink. Add salt and cumin and mix well. Cook for a few seconds.
4. Add beans and about a cup of water and mix well.
5. Lower the heat and cover with a lid. Cook for about 8-10 minutes.

6. Tear up a tortilla and spread on the bottom of the baking dish.
7. Spread half the beans over it followed by half the corn.
8. Spread half the vegan sour cream followed by half the salsa.
9. Repeat the layers one again(step 8-9)
10. Tear up the other tortillas and place on top. Spray the top layer of tortillas with cooking spray.
11. Cover the dish with foil and place it in the oven for 20 minutes.
12. Uncover and bake for some more time until crisp and brown on top.
13. Divide into two equal portions and serve with guacamole.

TUESDAY

BREAKFAST SWEET POTATO (BREAKFAST)

Nutritional values per serving:
One stuffed sweet potato

Number of servings: 3	**Calories:** 537	**Carbohydrate:** 45g	**Protein:** 20,7g
	Fat: 31g	**Fiber:** 9,4g	

Ingredients:

- 3 sweet potatoes (7 ounces each)
- 2 large eggs
- 2 slices bacon
- ½ small avocado, peeled, pitted chopped
- Salt to taste
- Garlic powder to taste
- Pepper to taste

Directions:

1. Set the temperature of the oven to 375°F and preheat the oven.
2. To bake sweet potatoes: Pierce holes all over the sweet potatoes using a fork and place it on a baking sheet.
3. Place the baking sheet in the oven and set the timer for 45-60 minutes or until fork tender.
4. Meanwhile, cook bacon until crisp. Remove bacon with a slotted spoon and place on a plate lined with paper towels. Crumble the bacon once it cools.
5. Retain a little bacon grease in the pan and drain off the rest.
6. Whisk together eggs with seasonings.
7. Pour eggs into the pan. Scramble them and cook to the desired doneness, stirring often.
8. Make a slit in the middle of the sweet potatoes and press the sides of the sweet potatoes to make space for stuffing.
9. Stuff the scrambled eggs, avocado and bacon (make sure you divide them equally) into the sweet potatoes and serve.

GREEK MEATBALLS (SNACK)

Number of servings:
8

Nutritional values per serving:
Four meatballs

Calories:	226	Carbohydrate:	3g	Protein:	34g
Fat:	9g	Fiber:	1g		

Ingredients:

- 2 2//3 pounds 95% lean ground beef or turkey
- Zest of two lemons, grated
- 4 cloves garlic, minced
- 2 teaspoons salt

- 1 teaspoon pepper
- ¼ teaspoon ground allspice
- 2 eggs
- ½ cup minced parsley
- 2 teaspoons oregano

- 1 teaspoon ground cumin
- 1 teaspoon ground coriander

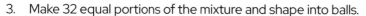

Directions:

1. Set the temperature of the oven to 375°F and preheat the oven. Prepare a baking sheet by spraying it with cooking spray.
2. Combine meat, lemon zest, salt, parsley, and spices in a bowl. Make sure it is just combined and not over-mixed else the meat will get tough.
3. Make 32 equal portions of the mixture and shape into balls.
4. Place the meatballs on the baking sheet and place it in the oven for 18-20 minutes. Make sure you do not bake them for long else the meatballs will become very dry.
5. Transfer onto a serving platter. Insert toothpicks in each meatball and serve.

ITALIAN LUNCH BOWLS (LUNCH)

	Nutritional values per serving:		
	One bowl		
Number of servings:	**Calories:** 376	**Carbohydrate:** 50g	**Protein:** 15g
3	**Fat:** 14g	**Fiber:** 8g	

Ingredients:

For bowls:

- 1 cup dry quinoa, soaked in water for 15 minutes, rinsed, drained
- ½ large cucumber, chopped
- 1 cup halved cherry tomatoes
- 2 cups water
- Thinly sliced green onion, to garnish
- ½ pound leafy greens of your choice like spinach, lettuce etc.
- ½–1 bell pepper of any color, deseeded, chopped
- 1–2 radishes, trimmed, thinly sliced
- 1 ½ cups cooked beans (optional)

For creamy Italian dressing:

- ¼ cup tahini
- ½ teaspoon apple cider vinegar
- 1 clove garlic, peeled
- ¼ teaspoon dried oregano
- ¼ cup water
- ¼ teaspoon salt
- 2 tablespoons fresh lemon juice
- ¼ teaspoon onion powder

Directions:

1. Cook quinoa and water in a saucepan over high heat. When it begins to boil, reduce the heat and cook until dry. Turn off the heat. Using a fork, fluff the quinoa.
2. Meanwhile, make the dressing by blending together all the ingredients of the dressing in a blender and blend until smooth.
3. Divide quinoa among three bowls. Divide the leafy greens and other vegetables and place over the quinoa. Spoon the dressing on top and serve.

GREEK SHRIMP SALAD WITH FETA AND RICE (DINNER)

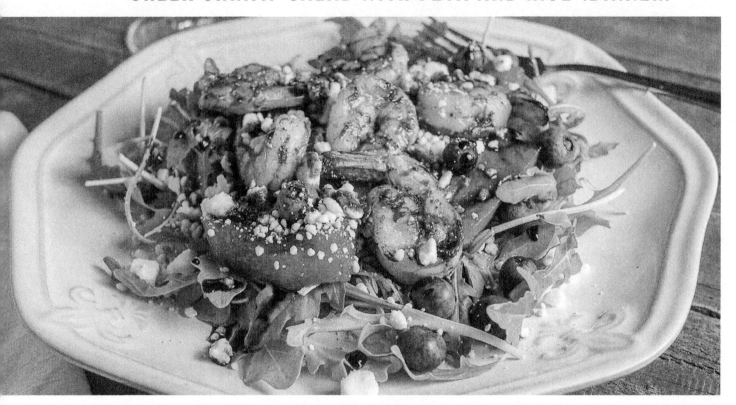

	Nutritional values per serving:		
Number of servings:	**Calories:** 407	**Carbohydrate:** 31g	**Protein:** 23g
3	**Fat:** 21g	**Fiber:** 3g	

Ingredients:

For salad:

- 2 cups cooked rice
- ½ cucumber, diced
- ½ pound medium shrimp, cooked
- ¼ cup chopped kalamata olives

- A large handful chopped parsley
- 1 tomato, deseeded, diced
- 1 ½ scallions, thinly sliced
- 3 ounces feta cheese, crumbled

For dressing:

- 1 clove garlic, peeled, minced
- 3 tablespoons olive oil
- Juice of a lemon or to taste
- ½ teaspoon salt

Directions:

1. To make salad: Combine rice, shrimp, parsley and vegetables in a bowl.
2. To make dressing: Whisk together oil, lemon juice, garlic, and salt in a bowl and pour over the salad.
3. Toss well.
4. Add feta and fold gently. Divide into three bowls and serve.

WEDNESDAY

SAVORY BREAKFAST BOWL (BREAKFAST)

Nutritional values per serving:
One bowl

Number of servings:	Calories:	654	Carbohydrate:	54g	Protein:	23g
2	Fat:	40g	Fiber:	13g		

Ingredients:

- 3 tablespoons olive oil
- 2 handfuls fresh baby spinach
- Pepper to taste
- 2 hard boiled eggs, peeled,
- quartered
- 2 small ripe avocados, peeled, pitted, thinly sliced
- 12 cherry tomatoes
- Salt to taste
- 2 cups cooked quinoa
- Black sesame seeds to garnish
- ½ cup cottage cheese

Directions:

1. Pour one tablespoon of oil into a skillet and place it over medium heat. When oil is hot, add spinach, tomatoes, salt, and pepper and cook for a couple of minutes until spinach wilts. Turn off the heat.
2. To assemble the bowls: Add one cup quinoa into each bowl. Add salt to taste and mix well.
3. Place eggs, avocado, and cottage cheese over the quinoa.
4. Layer with spinach and tomato mixture. Pour a tablespoon of oil on top in each bowl and serve.

EDAMAME CRUNCH (SNACK)

Nutritional values per serving:

Number of servings:	Calories:	115	Carbohydrate:	9,7g	Protein:	8,5g
2	Fat:	4,3g	Fiber:	4,5g		

Ingredients:

- 1 cup shelled edamame
- Salt to taste
- 2 teaspoons toasted sesame seeds

Directions:

1. Drop edamame into a pot of boiling water. Boil for a few minutes until crisp as well as tender.
2. Drain in a colander.
3. Divide edamame into two bowls. Add salt to taste and toss well. Garnish with sesame seeds and serve.

SUMMER STRAWBERRY CHICKEN SALAD (LUNCH)

	Nutritional values per serving:		
Number of servings: 2	**Calories:** 587 **Fat:** 31g	**Carbohydrate:** 43g **Fiber:** 11g	**Protein:** 39g

Ingredients:

For the salad:

- ½ pound chicken, cut
- Spices and herbs of your choice
- Olive oil to brush
- ½ avocado, peeled, pitted, sliced
- ¼ cup sliced strawberries
- 3 cups salad greens
- 1/8 cup crumbled goat cheese

For the dressing:

- ½ tablespoon olive oil
- ½ tablespoon lime juice
- ¼ cup full-fat Greek yogurt
- 1 tablespoon lemon juice
- 1 tablespoon honey

For strawberry marinade:

- ½ pound strawberries, sliced
- 1 tablespoon water
- 1 tablespoon coconut sugar
- ½ tablespoon lemon juice

Directions:

1. Set the temperature of the oven to 400°F and preheat the oven.
2. Brush oil over the chicken. Sprinkle spices and herbs of your choice over the chicken and place in a baking dish.
3. Place the baking dish in the oven and set the timing of the oven for 30 minutes or until the chicken is cooked. Turn the chicken half way through roasting.
4. Meanwhile, make the strawberry marinade: Combine strawberries, water, coconut sugar, and lemon juice in a pan. Place the pan over medium heat. When the mixture starts boiling, lower the heat and cook until thick like syrup.
5. Turn off the heat and transfer into a bowl. Add the grilled chicken and mix well. Let it sit for 10 minutes.
6. To assemble: Place salad greens, avocado, strawberries, and goat cheese in a bowl and toss well.
7. Divide the salad into two bowls or plates. Divide the chicken and place over the salad.
8. Serve.

CLAM CHOWDER (DINNER)

Nutritional values per serving:
11/3 cups

Number of servings:	Calories:	256	Carbohydrate:	33,4g	Protein:	12,1g
3	Fat:	9,53g	Fiber:	4,5g		

Ingredients:

- ¾ cup frozen corn, thawed
- 1 tablespoon extra-virgin olive oil
- ½ cup chopped onion
- 2 cloves garlic, minced
- 1 cup bottled clam juice
- 1 can (6.5 ounces)

- chopped clam, drained but retain the juice
- ¼ teaspoon pepper
- 1 strip bacon, chopped
- 1 cup chopped broccoli stems
- 1 ½ cups cubed potatoes

- 2 tablespoons whole-wheat or all-purpose flour
- ½ cup chicken broth
- 6 tablespoons half and half
- Salt to taste

Directions:

1. Dry the corn with paper towels. Place a soup pot over medium-high heat.
2. Add corn and cook until light brown. Do not stir until it turns light brown. Now stir and cook once again until light brown.
3. Remove corn into a bowl.
4. Add oil into the pot and let it heat. Add bacon and cook until crisp. Remove bacon with a slotted spoon and place on a plate lined with paper towels.
5. Add onion and broccoli stems and cook until a bit tender, 3-4 minutes.
6. Stir in garlic and potatoes and cook for about a minute. Add flour all over the vegetables and mix well. Stir for about a minute.
7. Add clam juice, retained juice, and broth. When the mixture starts boiling, lower the heat and cook covered until potatoes are cooked.
8. Add clam, pepper, bacon, corn, and half and half and heat for a couple of minutes.
9. Serve in bowls.

THURSDAY

PB AND J YOGURT PARFAIT (BREAKFAST)

	Nutritional values per serving: One glass				
Number of servings: 2	**Calories:**	315	**Carbohydrate:**	35,8g	**Protein:** 13g
	Fat:	14,3g	**Fiber:**	10,3g	

Ingredients:

- 1 cup plain Greek yogurt
- 2 teaspoons chia seeds
- 2 handfuls fresh berries of
- your choice
- 1/8 cup mixed nuts and seeds
- ½ teaspoon vanilla extract
- 2 tablespoons nut butter
- 4 tablespoons large oat flakes
- 2 tablespoons milk

Directions:

1. Combine chia seeds, vanilla, and yogurt in a bowl. Cover and keep it aside for a while for the chia seeds to swell up.
2. Take two parfait glasses and spread a tablespoon of nut butter on the bottom of the glasses.
3. Place a layer of chia seed mixture in the glasses. Place a layer of berries followed by oats.
4. Repeat the layers until the ingredients are used up.
5. Top with nuts. Drizzle a tablespoon of milk on top and serve.

TOMATO BASIL SKEWERS (SNACK)

	Nutritional values per serving: Four skewers				
Number of servings: 2	**Calories:**	184	**Carbohydrate:**	4g	**Protein:** 11,4g
	Fat:	13,2g	**Fiber:**	0,8g	

Ingredients:

- 8 small fresh mozzarella balls
- 8 cherry tomatoes
- Coarse salt to taste
- 8 fresh basil leaves
- Extra-virgin olive oil to drizzle
- Freshly ground pepper to taste

Directions:

1. Take eight small skewers or toothpicks. Build the skewers with one each of mozzarella, tomato and basil in each skewer.
2. Place the built skewers on a plate. Drizzle oil over the skewers. Season with salt and pepper and serve.

SALMON COUSCOUS SALAD (LUNCH)

	Nutritional values per serving: Four cups			
Number of servings: 2	**Calories:** 464	**Carbohydrate:** 34,7g	**Protein:** 34,8g	
	Fat: 22,1g	**Fiber:** 5,9g		

Ingredients:

- ½ cup sliced cremini mushrooms
- 6 cups baby spinach
- ½ cup cooked whole wheat Israeli couscous
- ½ cup chopped, dried apricots
- ½ cup diced eggplant
- 8 ounces cooked salmon
- 1 ounce goat cheese, crumbled

For white wine vinaigrette:
- 4 tablespoons white wine vinegar
- Salt to taste
- Pepper to taste
- ½ cup extra-virgin olive oil

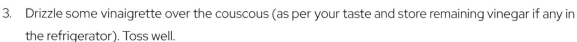

Directions:

1. Place a skillet over medium heat. Spray some cooking spray into the skillet. Add eggplant and mushroom and cook until light brown and some of the cooked juices are visible. Turn off the heat.
2. Place spinach in a bowl. Pour 2-3 tablespoons of the vinaigrette and toss well. Spread on a serving platter.
3. Drizzle some vinaigrette over the couscous (as per your taste and store remaining vinegar if any in the refrigerator). Toss well.
4. Spread couscous over the spinach. Next layer with salmon followed by cooked vegetables.
5. Scatter apricots and goat cheese on top and serve.

GARLIC BUTTER GROUND TURKEY WITH CAULIFLOWER SKILLET (DINNER)

	Nutritional values per serving:			
Number of servings:	**Calories:** 415,6	**Carbohydrate:** 16,3g	**Protein:** 30,65g
2	**Fat:** 26,11g	**Fiber:** 2,53g	

Ingredients:

- ½ pound ground turkey
- 1 tablespoon vegetable oil
- 1½ tablespoons butter
- ½ tablespoon onion powder
- 1 tablespoon hot sauce
- Chopped fresh cilantro or

- parsley to garnish
- Red chili flakes to taste
- ¼ head cauliflower, cut into florets, cooked
- ½ tablespoon lemon juice
- 1 tablespoon minced garlic

- 2 tablespoons soy sauce or coconut aminos
- 1/8 cup water
- Lemon slices to garnish

Directions:

1. Pour ½ tablespoon oil into a skillet and heat the skillet over medium-low heat.
2. When oil is hot, add cauliflower and cook until light brown. Turn off the heat. Transfer into a bowl.
3. Add lemon juice and stir. Add salt, pepper and cilantro and mix well.
4. Clean the skillet and place it over medium heat. Add butter and ½ tablespoon oil. When butter melts, add turkey and cook until it is not pink anymore. As you stir, break the meat into smaller pieces.
5. Stir in water, soy sauce, and hot sauce and cook for 2-3 minutes.
6. Add cauliflower and mix well. Heat thoroughly. Add red pepper flakes to taste
7. Serve with lemon slices.

FRIDAY

POACHED EGG BUDDHA BOWLS (BREAKFAST)

Nutritional values per serving:

Number of servings:	Calories:	526	Carbohydrate:	58g	Protein:	21g
1	Fat:	24g	Fiber:	10g		

Ingredients:

- ¼ cup + 1/8 cup wheat berries
- 1 ¼ cups water
- 1 tablespoon fresh lemon juice
- Salt to taste
- ¼ cup quartered cherry tomatoes
- 1 tablespoon sliced Greek olives
- ¼ cup low-fat ricotta cheese
- 1 large egg
- 1 tablespoon olive oil + extra to drizzle
- ½ tablespoon thinly sliced fresh mint leaves
- Freshly ground pepper to taste

Directions:

1. Combine water and wheat berries in a saucepan. Place the saucepan over medium heat. When it starts boiling, lower the heat and cover with a lid. Cook until soft.
2. Meanwhile, place a pan filled with water over medium heat. When water starts boiling, crack an egg into a bowl and slide it into the pan. Cook until the whites are set. Remove with a slotted spoon and place on a plate lined with paper towels.
3. Drain into a colander and allow it to cool for a few minutes. Transfer into a bowl.
4. Add oil, salt, pepper, and lemon juice and mix well.
5. Scatter tomatoes, olives and ricotta cheese on top. Place the egg right on top. Season with salt and pepper and serve.

HUMMUS BELL PEPPER AND FETA CRACKERS (SNACK)

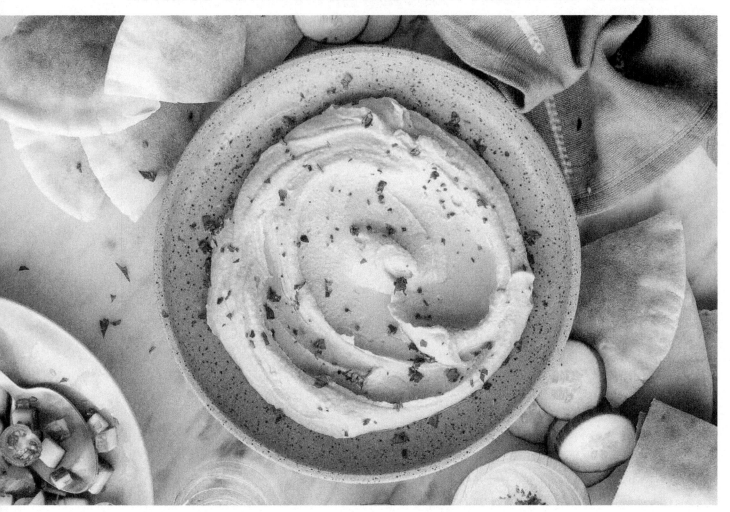

	Nutritional values per serving:				
	**Calories:**	136	**Carbohydrate:**	13,1g	**Protein:**
Number of servings:	**Fat:**	1,7g	**Fiber:**	3,6g	
2					6g

Ingredients:

- 4 tablespoons hummus
- ¼ cup crumbled feta cheese

- 2 large whole-grain crispbread like Wasa sourdough whole-grain crispbread

- ¼ cup diced bell peppers

Directions:

1. Spread two tablespoons of hummus on each crispbread. Scatter feta cheese and bell pepper on top and serve.

SHRIMP TACOS (LUNCH)

Nutritional values per serving:
Three tacos

| **Number of servings:** 2 | **Calories:** 492 | **Carbohydrate:** 32g | **Protein:** 43g |
| | **Fat:** 22g | **Fiber:** 4g | |

Ingredients:

- ¾ pound raw shrimp, peeled, deveined, remove tail
- Juice of ½ lime
- ½ teaspoon ground cumin
- 2 small cloves garlic, minced
- ½ tablespoon olive oil
- ½ teaspoon chili powder

- ¼ teaspoon paprika
- 1/8 teaspoon cayenne pepper or to taste

For sauce:
- 6 tablespoons plain Greek yogurt
- 1 teaspoon white vinegar
- ¼ jalapeño pepper, sliced
- A pinch onion powder

- 2 tablespoons olive oil
- ½ clove garlic, minced
- 1/8 cup chopped cilantro
- ¼ teaspoon salt

To serve:
- 6 small corn tortillas
- 1 cup finely shredded cabbage

Directions:

1. Dry the shrimp by patting with paper towels. Place shrimp in a bowl. Drizzle oil, spices, and lime juice and toss well. Cover and chill until use.
2. Meanwhile, make the taco sauce by blending together yogurt, vinegar, pepper, oil, cilantro, onion powder, garlic, salt, and cilantro.
3. Pour into a bowl. Cover and keep it refrigerated until use.
4. Place a skillet over medium-high heat. Add oil and let it heat. Once oil is hot, add shrimp and cook for a couple of minutes on each side until pink and cooked as well.
5. To make slaw: Combine cabbage with half the sauce mixture.
6. To build the tacos: Divide the shrimp among the tortillas. Divide the slaw as well.
7. Scatter avocado on top. Spoon the remaining sauce on top and serve.

CREAMY CHICKEN ENCHILADA SOUP (DINNER)

	Nutritional values per serving:		
Number of servings:	**Calories:** 450	**Carbohydrate:** 52g	**Protein:** 34g
3	**Fat:** 13g	**Fiber:** 15g	

Ingredients:

- ½ tablespoon butter or avocado oil
- 1 stalk celery, sliced
- ½ large red bell pepper, diced
- ¾ teaspoon ground cumin
- ½ teaspoon dried oregano
- 2 tablespoons tomato paste
- ½ can (from a 15.5 ounces can) red kidney beans, drained, rinsed
- ½ cup fresh or frozen sweet corn
- ½ cup Mexican cheese blend
- ½ medium onion, diced
- ½ medium carrot, thinly sliced
- 2 cloves garlic, peeled, chopped
- ½ tablespoon chili powder
- ½ can (from a 15 ounces can) diced fire-roasted
- tomatoes
- 2 cups low sodium chicken broth
- ½ can (from a 15.5 ounces can) black beans, drained, rinsed
- 1 cup cooked, shredded chicken
- Salt to taste
- Pepper to taste

Directions:

1. Pour oil into a soup pot and heat it over medium-high heat. When oil is hot, add celery, onion, bell pepper, carrot, and garlic and mix well. Cook until the vegetables are tender.
2. Add tomatoes, broth, tomato paste, salt, and spices and mix well. Reduce the heat and simmer until vegetables are cooked. Turn off the heat.
3. Blend the mixture with an immersion blender until smooth.
4. Add red beans, black beans, chicken, and corn and heat the soup thoroughly.
5. Ladle into soup bowls. Garnish with cheese and serve.

SATURDAY

CINNAMON QUINOA BREAKFAST BOWL (BREAKFAST)

Nutritional values per serving:
Onebowl

Number of servings:	**Calories:**	450	**Carbohydrate:**	68g	**Protein:**	12g
2	**Fat:**	16g	**Fiber:**	9g		

Ingredients:

For quinoa:

- ½ cup quinoa, rinsed, drained
- 1 teaspoon ground cinnamon
- 1/8 teaspoon sea salt
- 1 ½ cups almond milk
- 1 teaspoon vanilla extract

For toppings:

- 2 bananas, sliced
- 2 tablespoons shredded coconut
- ¼ cup chopped almonds
- 2 teaspoons maple syrup

Directions:

1. Combine quinoa, cinnamon, almond milk, salt, and vanilla in a saucepan. Place the saucepan over medium heat.
2. When the mixture begins to boil, lower the heat and simmer until nearly dry. Turn off the heat.
3. Divide the quinoa into two bowls. Place banana slices, coconut and almonds on top.
4. Trickle a teaspoon of maple syrup on top in each bowl and serve.

FIG AND RICOTTA TOAST (SNACK)

Number of servings: 2	Nutritional values per serving: One toast					
	Calories:	252	**Carbohydrate:**	32,1g	**Protein:**	12,5g
	Fat:	9,1g	**Fiber:**	4,3g		

Ingredients:

- 2 slices crusty whole-grain bread, toasted
- 2 fresh figs or four dried figs, sliced
- 2 teaspoons honey
- ½ cup part-skim ricotta cheese
- 2 teaspoons toasted, sliced almonds
- A large pinch flaky sea saltc

Directions:

1. Spread four tablespoons of part-skim ricotta cheese on each toast. Place fig slices over the toast.
2. Scatter almonds on the toast. Sprinkle flaky sea salt on top and serve.

WATERMELON OLIVE SALAD (LUNCH)

Number of servings: 2	Nutritional values per serving:					
	Calories:	352	**Carbohydrate:**	27g	**Protein:**	8g
	Fat:	26g	**Fiber:**	7g		

Ingredients:

- 3 cups cubed watermelon
- 2 ounces feta cheese, crumbled
- 1 tablespoon olive oil
- 4 ounces pitted black kalamata olives
- 10 mint leaves, thinly sliced
- Salt to taste
- Black pepper to taste

Directions:

1. Place watermelon, olives, mint leaves, and feta cheese in a bowl and toss well.
2. Drizzle oil, salt, and pepper and toss well.
3. Divide into two bowls and serve.

LENTIL AND MUSHROOM STEW OVER POTATO PARSNIP MASH (DINNER)

Nutritional values per serving:

Number of servings:	Calories:	470	Carbohydrate:	66g	Protein:	15g
2	Fat:	16g	Fiber:	15g		

Ingredients:

For parsnip and potato mash:

- ½ tablespoon parsnip, peeled
- ½ pound Yukon gold potatoes or russet potatoes, partially peeled
- 1 tablespoon butter
- ¼ cup milk of your choice
- Salt to taste
- 1 teaspoon chopped fresh rosemary

For stew:

- 1 tablespoon olive oil
- 4 ounces shiitake mushrooms
- 4 ounces cremini mushrooms, sliced
- ½ yellow onion, finely chopped
- 2 cloves garlic, minced
- ¼ cup dry red wine
- 3 thyme sprigs
- ½ teaspoon black pepper

or to taste

- 1 tablespoon flour
- 1 tablespoon low sodium soy sauce or tamari
- 1½ tablespoons tomato paste
- ½ tablespoon chopped fresh rosemary
- Salt to taste
- 1 cup vegetable broth
- ½ cup cooked or canned brown lentils

Directions:

1. To make parsnip and potato mash: Cook potatoes and parsnip in a pot of water with a little salt, until soft.
2. Drain and place in a bowl. Mash with a potato masher. Stir in milk, butter, salt, and pepper. Cover and keep warm.
3. While the vegetables are cooking, make the stew: Pour oil into a skillet and heat it over medium-high heat.
4. When oil is hot, add onion and mushrooms and cook until mushrooms turn brown.
5. Stir in tomato paste and garlic and cook until thick.
6. Stir in wine, salt, pepper, and herbs and cook until wine cooks down to half its original quantity.
7. Add flour, broth, and soy sauce and keep stirring until the stew is thick.
8. Add lentils and stir. Discard the thyme sprigs.
9. Divide the mash among two serving bowls. Divide the stew equally and pour over the mash.

S U N D A Y

TURKEY CHILI SHAKSHUKA (BREAKFAST)

Nutritional values per serving:

Number of servings:	Calories:	515	Carbohydrate:	43g	Protein:	38g
3	Fat:	22g	Fiber:	14g		

Ingredients:

- ½ pound ground turkey
- ½ orange bell pepper, diced
- ½ tablespoon olive oil
- ½ can (from a 15.5 ounces can) black beans
- ½ can (from a 15.5 ounces can) pinto beans
- ½ onion, chopped
- 1 cloves garlic, peeled,

- minced
- ½ can (from a 28 ounces can) peeled diced tomatoes
- 2 eggs
- A handful fresh cilantro, chopped
- 1 teaspoon chili powder
- Salt to taste

- ½ teaspoon ground cumin
- ¼ teaspoon crushed red pepper or to taste
- Low-fat sour cream to garnish
- ¼ cup grated cheddar cheese
- Sliced green chilies to taste

Directions:

1. Pour oil into a heavy bottomed, ovenproof skillet and heat it over medium flame.
2. Add turkey, onion, garlic, green chili, and bell pepper and cook until the meat is cooked.
3. Stir in the tomatoes, salt, spices and beans. Let it come to a rolling boil. Lower the heat to low heat and cook for another 10 minutes. Stir often.
4. Make two cavities in the mixture. Crack an egg into each cavity. Cook until the eggs are cooked for five minutes. Turn off the heat.
5. Meanwhile, set your oven to broil mode and preheat the oven.
6. Shift the skillet into the oven and broil for two minutes. Sprinkle cheese on top and broil for another 2-3 minutes.
7. Drizzle sour cream on top and serve.

CLEMENTINE AND PISTACHIO RICOTTA (SNACK)

Nutritional values per serving:

Number of servings:	Calories:	356	Carbohydrate:	29,2g	Protein:	22,2g
1	Fat:	18g	Fiber:	3,6g		

Ingredients:

- 2/3 cup part-skim ricotta cheese
- 4 teaspoons chopped pistachios
- 2 clementine's, peeled, separated into segments

Directions:

1. Place ricotta cheese in each bowl.
2. Add clementine segments and stir. Garnish with two teaspoons of pistachios on top, in each bowl and serve.

BALSAMIC PORK AND STRAWBERRY SALAD (LUNCH)

	Nutritional values per serving:		
	Three ounces cooked pork with 1 ½ cups salad		
Number of servings:	**Calories:** 278	**Carbohydrate:** 12,6g	**Protein:** 28,5g
2	**Fat:** 11,7g	**Fiber:** 2,5g	

Ingredients:

- ½ pound pork tenderloin, trimmed of fat
- 1 tablespoon Dijon mustard
- 1/8 teaspoon salt or to taste
- 2 cups torn lettuce leaves

- 1 ounce shredded Manchego cheese
- ¼ cup balsamic vinegar
- ½ tablespoon olive oil
- 1/8 teaspoon black pepper

- or to taste
- 1 cup quartered fresh strawberries

Directions:

1. To make marinade: Combine vinegar and mustard in a bowl. Pour 1 ½ tablespoons of marinade into a bowl and keep it aside.
2. Add meat into the remaining vinegar mixture. Turn the meat around in the bowl to coat it well.
3. Cover the bowl and chill for 15 minutes.
4. Set the temperature of the oven to 425°F and preheat the oven. Prepare a roasting pan by lining it with foil.
5. Take out the meat from the marinade and place it in the roasting pan. The marinade is to be discarded.
6. Place the roasting pan in the oven and roast until the internal temperature of the meat in the thickest part shows 145°F on the meat thermometer.
7. Take out the roasting pan from the oven and let it rest for five minutes. Cut the meat into slices.
8. To make salad: Combine the retained marinade, salt, pepper, and oil.
9. Combine strawberries and lettuce in a bowl.
10. Divide the salad among two serving plates. Scatter cheese on top.
11. Place meat slices on top and serve.

SKILLET BEEF POT PIE WITH BUTTERMILK BISCUITS (DINNER)

Nutritional values per serving:
1½ cups

Number of servings:	Calories:	420	Carbohydrate:	35,8g	Protein:	25,5g
2	Fat:	19,3g	Fiber:	6,7g		

Ingredients:

- ½ tablespoon extra-virgin olive oil
- 2 cloves garlic, minced
- Salt to taste
- 6.5 ounces frozen peas
- ½ cup +1 ½ tablespoons white whole-wheat flour, divided
- ¼ cup chopped parsley + extra to garnish
- 2 tablespoons unsalted butter, cut into ¼ inch pieces
- ½ pound lean ground beef
- ½ tablespoon Dijon mustard
- ½ bag (from a 14 ounces bag) pearl onions
- ½ cup diced carrots
- 1 ½ cups low-sodium beef broth
- ¼ teaspoon baking powder
- ¼ cup buttermilk

Directions:

1. Set the temperature of the oven to 400°F and preheat the oven.
2. Pour oil into an ovenproof skillet and place it over medium-high heat.
3. When oil is hot, add beef and cook until brown. As you stir, make sure to break the meat into pieces.
4. Stir in garlic, salt, and mustard. Keep stirring for a minute.
5. Add carrots, peas, and onions and mix well. Stir often until the mixture is thoroughly heated.
6. Dust 1 ½ tablespoons flour over the mixture and mix well for about a minute.
7. Stir in broth. Keep stirring until a bit thick.
8. Add parsley and mix well. Turn off the heat.
9. Place remaining flour in a bowl. Add baking powder and a pinch of salt and mix well.
10. Scatter butter over the mixture and cut the butter into the flour until sand-like in texture.
11. Add buttermilk and stir until just incorporated. Drop heaping tablespoonfuls of the batter (this is one biscuit) over the beef. You should be able to get six biscuits in all.
12. Shift the skillet into the oven. Set the timing for about 20 minutes. Bake until golden brown on top.
13. Sprinkle parsley on top and serve.

CONCLUSION AND GIFT!

I want to thank you once again for choosing this book. I hope it proved to be an enjoyable and informative read.

Following the Mediterranean diet is not complicated. It is not a restrictive diet and instead, includes a variety of fresh and wholesome ingredients rich in nutrients without any unhealthy or harmful calories. The first step to improve your health is by paying attention to your diet. From losing weight and maintaining it to reducing the risk of chronic diseases, the Mediterranean diet offers several advantages. Also, this diet is perfectly sustainable in the long run. It is a celebration of delicious food and life.

All the recipes given in this book are designed to make cooking delicious and healthy meals easy. Don't forget to use the sample meal plan while shifting to this diet. By eliminating processed and refined foods from your diet and replacing them with wholesome ingredients, you can attain all the benefits it offers. Once you start following this diet, you will see a positive change. In the meanwhile, be a little patient and believe in this diet.

By following the simple protocols of the Mediterranean diet, you will essentially be eating your way to a healthier and fitter life! Now, all you need to do is simply follow the suggestions given in this book to get started with this diet! The key to your health and fitness lies in your hands. Take the first up today and shift to the Mediterranean way of living.

Thank you and all the best!

"Thank you for reading This book."

If you enjoyed it, please visit the site where you purchased it and write a brief review. Your feedback is important to me.

Want More? Do you want even more recipes?
DOWNLOAD 200 RECIPES FOR FREE HERE

FOLLOW ME!

Printed in Great Britain
by Amazon